Social Work, Law and Ethics

Law and ethics are two vital aspects of social work – all social workers need to practise according to the law and their codes of ethics and conduct. However, the relationship between the law and social work values and ethics is not without its tensions and this book takes a problem-based approach to explore the dilemmas and challenges that can arise.

The first part of the book sets out frameworks for thinking about the law and ethics, and how they relate to social work. It also introduces some of the big philosophical and sociological questions about the purposes of law and of ethics and how they relate to society more generally.

The second part explores a series of areas where profound dilemmas arise – such as end of life decisions, respecting people's choices but ensuring their safety and that of others, responsibility and blame, making allowance for different cultural traditions and breaking confidentiality. In each of the problem-based chapters, this accessible text:

- outlines the relevant law;
- discusses court judgments in leading cases;
- considers the implications of different ethical frameworks;
- pulls out key ethical questions and challenges for social work.

Social Work, Law and Ethics highlights what the law says and what it offers, which ethical principles are at stake, and what these imply for social work policy and practice. In this way, it uses real-life scenarios to analyse the dynamic interactions of social work, law and ethics. It is essential reading for all social work students.

Jonathan Dickens is Senior Lecturer in Social Work at the University of East Anglia, UK. He is the author of another book in the Routledge Student Social Work series, *Social Work and Social Policy: An introduction.*

Student Social Work

This exciting new textbook series is ideal for all students studying to be qualified social workers, whether at undergraduate or masters level. Covering key elements of the social work curriculum, the books are accessible, interactive and thought-provoking.

New titles

Human Growth and Development
John Sudbery

Mental Health Social Work in Context
Nick Gould

Social Work and Social Policy
An introduction
Jonathan Dickens

Social Work Placements
Mark Doel

Social Work
A reader
Viviene E. Cree

Sociology for Social Workers and Probation Officers
Viviene E. Cree

Integrating Social Work Theory and Practice
A practical skills guide
Pam Green Lister

Social Work, Law and Ethics
Jonathan Dickens

Forthcoming titles

Social Work with Children and Young People, their Families and Carers
Janet Warren

Becoming a Social Worker, 2nd edn
Narratives from around the world
Viviene E. Cree

Social Work, Law and Ethics

Jonathan Dickens

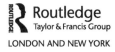
Routledge
Taylor & Francis Group

LONDON AND NEW YORK

First published 2013
by Routledge
2 Park Square, Milton Park, Abingdon, Oxon, OX14 4RN

Simultaneously published in the USA and Canada
by Routledge
711 Third Avenue, New York, NY 10017

Routledge is an imprint of the Taylor & Francis Group, an informa business

British Library Cataloguing in Publication Data
A catalogue record for this book is available from the British Library

Library of Congress Cataloging-in-Publication Data
Dickens, Jonathan, 1961-
Social work, law and ethics / Jonathan Dickens.
p. cm. — (Student social work)
1. Social service. 2. Social workers—Legal status, laws, etc. 3. Social workers—Professional ethics.
I. Title.
HV40.35.D534 2013
174'.9361–dc23
2012011897

ISBN13: 978-0-415-59015-0 (hbk)
ISBN13: 978-0-415-59016-7 (pbk)
ISBN13: 978-0-203-09506-5 (ebk)

Typeset in Rotis by
Keystroke, Station Road, Codsall, Wolverhampton

Contents

Boxes and tables

Boxes

Tables

Cases

Acknowledgements

Thanks to colleagues in the School of Social Work at the University of East Anglia for their helpful comments on draft chapters: Ann McDonald, Carol Dawson, Marian Brandon, David Howe, Chris Beckett and Nigel Stone. Any mistakes that remain are, of course, my responsibility. I would especially like to acknowledge the advice and encouragement of Ann McDonald and Carol Dawson. The three of us have shared the teaching of law to social work students at the University of East Anglia for many years now, and I have benefited from their knowledge and enthusiasm about the subject and how to help students learn it. I have also been fortunate to co-teach a course on values in social work with Roger Hennessey, and learned a lot from his understandings and insights. As always, thanks and love to Julia and Caitlin.

Introduction

What's the right thing to do? For social workers the question has an extra-sharp edge. What's the right thing to do in this particular case, with this particular family, this service user? Sometimes it can seem as though there are many different answers to the question, and certainly there are very many places to look for an answer. There are our agency's policies and procedures, the wishes of the service users, our assessment of their needs, our own personal values, our professional codes, government regulations and the laws of the land. Finding a way through this forest can be a daunting task.

The aim of this book is to focus on two of the most important places that social workers need to look when they are trying to find an answer to that hard question, the right thing to do: law and ethics. Many of the roles and tasks that social workers undertake are set out in legislation, and all of them are covered by ethics. There has been a long-running debate in social work about the relationship between law and ethics – which is on top, and how they interact. Both are essential, but saying that is only the starting point, because then we need to think about how they relate to one another, what happens when they clash, and how they link with other driving forces in contemporary practice, notably budgets and organisational priorities. Knowledge and understanding of the law and of ethics are two of the key responsibilities for social workers. They are something that social workers are expected to continue learning about and developing in, right through their careers. I hope that this book will help as a foundation and framework for that.

The book focuses on social work law, policy and practice in England, although reference is made to the other countries of the United Kingdom as appropriate. Social work is one of the policy areas that is dealt with by the separate countries (England, Wales, Scotland and Northern Ireland), but within an overall framework of UK legislation and policy (headed by the Houses of Parliament and the UK Supreme Court - see Chapter 3). There are differences of law and policy between the four countries, but social workers face similar challenges in all of them (Dickens, 2012). The focus may be England but the book is always trying to find and apply general principles - for example, about justice, duty, fairness, freedom, choice and so on - and so I hope that readers in other countries will find material of interest, and ideas that are helpful.

The context

Over the time that I was writing this book, 2010 to 2012, social work in England was undergoing a major period of scrutiny and change. It is certainly not the first time that it has experienced such a process, and nor will it be the last (Dickens, 2011), but it does leave social workers at the moment in a situation of particular uncertainty. Four aspects are especially relevant to the themes of law and ethics.

The GSCC and the code of practice for social care workers

First, the regulatory body, the General Social Care Council (GSCC), was abolished in summer 2012 and its functions transferred to the Health Professions Council (HPC), which was renamed the Health and Care Professions Council (HCPC). The HPC regulated a number of health and allied professions such as physiotherapists, occupational therapists, paramedics, chiropodists and dieticians (doctors and nurses have their own organisations). The GSCC regulated social work education, maintained a register of qualified social workers and social work students, and promoted high standards of conduct through its codes of practice for social care workers and employers (GSCC, 2002a). The code for employers was never made compulsory, but social workers had to comply with the workers' code and could be suspended or removed from the register if they breached it. The code was replaced by the HPC's standards of conduct, performance and ethics (HPC, 2008), and it is proposed that in due course they will be revised to take account of the arrival of social workers. The social care code remains in force for social workers in Scotland, Wales and Northern Ireland. The social care regulatory bodies there remain in existence (the Scottish Social Services Council, the Care Council for Wales and the Northern Ireland Social Care Council).

BASW and the code of ethics for social work

Second, the place of the leading professional association for the last forty years, the British Association of Social Workers (BASW), has been unsettled by government-backed plans to establish a College of Social Work. Membership of BASW has never been compulsory and the large majority of social workers in the UK do not belong. However, it has been the largest professional body and has had an influential voice in the on-going debates about the role and the future of social work.

The proposal for a professional college to promote social work (as distinct from a regulator, like the GSCC) came from the Social Work Task Force in 2009. This had been set up by the Labour government in late 2008, in the wake of the national outcry about the death of 'Baby Peter' (Peter Connelly – discussed further in Chapter 9). Its task was to advise the government on a comprehensive reform programme for social work in children's and adult services. It produced three reports in 2009 (SWTF, 2009a, 2009b, 2009c). The work was then passed on to a new body, the Social Work Reform Board (SWRB, 2010). This took forward the plans for a professional college. There have been very difficult discussions between BASW and the College over the last two years about whether or not they will combine, the terms of any merger, and the independence and objectives of the new body.

BASW first published a code of ethics for social work in 1975. It was revised in 1986, to give greater weight to anti-oppressive values, and again in 2002, to enhance the human rights dimensions. In October 2011 BASW launched a consultation on a draft revision, to take account of new under-standings of social work and the challenges that social workers face. The final version of the new code was published in January 2012. References to the BASW code in this book are to the 2012 version, but there are substantial continuities between the previous version and the new one (BASW, 2002, 2012). The new code draws heavily on the international statement of ethical principles in social work, adopted in 2004 by the International Federation of Social Workers and the International Association of Schools of Social Work (IFSW and IASSW, 2004).

The international statement and the BASW code emphasise three key dimensions of social work ethics: human rights, social justice and professional conduct (the BASW code uses the term 'professional integrity'). The BASW code highlights three ways that ethical dilemmas can often arise for social workers (BASW, 2012: 6):

• dealing with conflicting interests and competing rights;

• having a role to support and empower people, alongside statutory duties and other obligations that may be coercive and restrict people's freedoms;

• being constrained by limited resources and organisational policies.

The case examples discussed in this book show the realities of those dilemmas.

Social work education and the professional capabilities framework

The Social Work Task Force also recommended changes to social work education, at qualifying and post-qualifying levels. Again, this was taken forward by the Social Work Reform Board and in December 2010 it produced a new framework for professional standards (SWRB, 2010). This features nine essential capabilities, which apply (at different levels) at all stages of a social worker's career, right from initial training through to advanced practice and managerial posts. The idea is that social workers must be able to demonstrate skill and understanding in each of these nine areas, as appropriate to their level of experience and their post, and keep developing them throughout their careers. The nine capabilities are:

- *professionalism* (e.g. to behave with professional integrity at all times);

- *values and ethics* (e.g. to engage in ethical decision-making and to know about the value base of the profession);

- *diversity* (e.g. to respect the diversity of human identity and experience, and appropriately challenge oppression);

- *rights, justice and economic well-being* (e.g. to recognise the fundamental principles of human rights and apply these in practice);

- *knowledge* (e.g. to understand human development and the law, and be able to apply this knowledge in practice);

- *critical reflection and analysis* (e.g. able to assess multiple sources of knowledge and evidence, able to think clearly and creatively);

- *intervention and skills* (e.g. able to use professional judgment and communication skills, able to use authority appropriately);

- *contexts and organisations* (e.g. able to work effectively as members of their own organisation, and able to work in multi-agency and inter-professional settings)

- *professional leadership* (e.g. to assist in the learning and development of others).

Social work degrees and post-qualifying courses in England will be revised over the next few years to take account of the new professional capabilities framework. It is clear that ethics and the law remain as important as ever. The challenge is to integrate knowledge and skill in ethics and the law with other fields of knowledge and other types of skill, and develop the ability to apply ethical and legal reasoning in practice, wisely and sensitively.

Policy changes and law reforms

There is also a fast-moving policy context, particularly in the light of the change of government in May 2010 and on-going economic difficulties. In children and families social work a key development has been that the Conservative–Liberal Democrat coalition government commissioned Professor Eileen Munro to lead a review of child protection, which recommended a reduction in overly detailed prescription and bureaucracy, and greater room for professional judgment (Munro, 2010, 2011a, 2011b). This will require new approaches to the selection, education, support and supervision of staff. Munro also recommended a refreshed emphasis on early intervention in families to prevent problems arising, a theme that has been echoed in other policy reviews (e.g. Field, 2010; Allen, 2011).

In adult social care, the theme of greater personalisation of services continues from the previous government, and the Law Commission finished its review of adult care law (Law Commission, 2008, 2010, 2011). The coalition commissioned a new enquiry into the funding of long-term care ('the Dilnot report': Commission on Funding of Care and Support, 2011), and is also planning major changes to welfare benefits that are likely to have a significant impact on those who require long-term support. Calls for clearer legislation, better funding and closer integration of health and social care are nothing new, but have been repeated by the House of Commons Health Committee (2012). Funding cut-backs to local authorities are having an increasingly severe impact on their ability to provide preventive services, as they restrict their spending to only those in the highest levels of need. In the light of all these changes, a white paper on adult social care was due in summer 2012.

The book

Given all these developments, I try in this book, as far as possible, to go back to first principles about ethics and the law, and then show how the big questions and the enduring themes are played out in current practice, by discussing real cases and social work dilemmas.

There are many excellent books about social work law, and about social work values and ethics. This book is not an alternative to those more specialist texts. It does not try to cover all the relevant law, or all the ethical theories, but rather takes certain aspects to illustrate and explore key debates about fairness, freedom, responsibility, proper decision-making, the role of social workers and the state. So, readers will need to refer to other books, journal articles and specialist websites, and I hope the references and suggestions for further reading will help with that. Also, when faced with a particular problem, readers will need to get up-to-date legal and professional advice. The law is continually changing, through new legislation and new court judgments, and ethical understandings are always moving on.

The purpose of the book, then, as stated earlier, is to be a foundation and framework for exploring the links between law, ethics and social work. Three dimensions are crucial for doing this:

- first, to appreciate the *dynamic interaction* of law, ethics and social work practice, with no simple or fixed answers;

- second, to see this in the *broader context* of social policies, social values and bigger questions about the purposes of law, the purposes of ethics and the purposes of social work;

- third, to look at the *practical implications*, the specific issues that arise for social workers in putting law and values into practice.

These are the guiding themes for this book. The first part (Chapters 1 to 5) sets out the key principles and frameworks.

Chapter 1 introduces the main themes by giving some historical background from the 1980s, and by setting out four key aspects of tension and ambiguity: between rights and responsibilities, freedom and control, the individual and society, the quest for certainty and the reality of uncertainty.

Chapter 2 explores the notion of fairness, by unpicking the complexities of justice, equality, human rights and the 'duty of care'.

Chapter 3 outlines the legal framework in England and Wales, describing the court structure and different types of law, the importance of politics and the principles of lawful decision-making.

Chapter 4 sets out four understandings of ethics: that doing the right thing means doing one's categorical duty (Kantianism), or doing whatever brings the best consequences (utilitarianism), or acting in good character (virtue ethics), or demonstrating care for the other person (care ethics). It also draws out the tensions between reason and emotion as mainsprings of ethical conduct.

Chapter 5 looks at the issues from another perspective, in terms of four freedoms: freedom from undue state control, freedom from inequality and oppression, freedom for all to enjoy their own culture, and freedom for individuals to be authentic. It also discusses two vital questions about the role of law in society, namely whether it is of primary or secondary importance in maintaining social order, and whether it serves the general welfare or the interests of the rich and powerful.

The second part of the book (Chapters 6 to 13) applies the concepts to social work law, policy and practice, using real life cases to illustrate and develop the themes.

Chapters 6 and 7 explore the limitations and realities of 'choice'. Freedom and choice are fundamental values in our society, and central to modern ideas about social work, but what happens in the hardest cases? Chapter 6 considers this with regard to end of life decisions, namely withdrawing life-sustaining treatment from a disabled child, and assisted suicide. Chapter 7 discusses issues of choice and risk in relation to the concepts of mental capacity (for adults) and 'Gillick competence' (for children and young people).

Chapters 8 and 9 are another pair, which explore different aspects of responsibility in social work, using child safeguarding work to illustrate the dilemmas. Chapter 8 discusses the challenges of protecting children whilst respecting and supporting parents' rights and responsibilities, and making allowance for difficult circumstances. Chapter 9 discusses the dilemmas of social workers' responsibilities and whether they should be blamed for bad outcomes.

Chapter 10 looks at crime, punishment and protection. It discusses the various principles of punishment and the tensions between them, and the challenges of achieving effective and fair public protection.

Chapter 11 explores some of the challenges of putting social work's anti-oppressive principles into practice. A core theme in social work values is to respect cultural, ethnic and lifestyle differences, but the two issues discussed in this chapter, mental health and forced marriages, reveal gaps between the rhetoric and the reality, and the challenges of ensuring equality and safety for all.

Chapter 12 investigates the tensions between principles of confidentiality and requirements to share information for service users' well-being and protection. It also discusses recent developments to allow journalists to publish anonymised reports on cases in the welfare courts, as an example of the tensions between privacy and openness.

Chapter 13 considers the nature of individual responsibility in organisational settings. It discusses whistleblowing, professional boundaries, organisational culture and resource limitations. It ends the book by arguing that despite the great organisational pressures – in fact, *because* of them – it is vital for social workers to retain a strong sense of personal responsibility and integrity, with an active, critical awareness of the requirements of the law and the underlying ethics of social work.

Each of the chapters has questions for reflection. I hope these will be useful to guide personal thinking, group discussions and further research. The chapters end with a list of useful websites and suggestions for further reading. Full reference details of the books are in the bibliography.

Part I Principles and frameworks

1 Key concepts

This book is driven by two central questions:

- What are the roles of law and ethics in social work, and how can we understand the relationship between them?

- How can social workers strike the right balances between promoting the rights and independence of service users, whilst protecting them and others from harm?

These are perennial questions, coming up time and again throughout the history of social work and as pertinent today as ever. Box 1.1 gives an introduction to the issues as they arose in the 1980s, when the arguments became especially heated. Since then the role of the law in social work in England has become much more prominent, and the ethical dimensions have changed a great deal too, with much more explicit attention to themes of empowerment and anti-oppressive practice: but the fundamental challenge remains – what's the best approach to helping people *and* protecting them and others?

In recent years in England the debates have become heated once again. Partly this is because of two child abuse deaths, the cases of Victoria Climbié (died in 2000: report of the inquiry, Laming, 2003) and

Chapter 9

'Baby Peter' (died in 2007: Haringey LSCB, 2009; Laming, 2009 – discussed in Chapter 9). These have brought much criticism of social work and (some) calls for more assertive, questioning and controlling approaches to service users. Alongside these developments, there have been considerable changes in the field of adult social care. Here, the emphasis is on giving greater choice and control to service users, raising hard questions about how to balance this with safety (of the service user and others), equity (how does one weigh the wishes and interests of different people?) and best use of limited resources.

These developments have brought social work in England to a very testing period of change and reform, as discussed in the Introduction. In this context, it is important to look back to first principles, to identify and hold on to what is distinctive and valuable about the profession. To do this we need to go back to the law and to ethics, two of social work's foundation stones.

There are differences between law and ethics as the discussion in Box 1.1 shows. But there are also similarities. Both address the profound challenges of reconciling individual conduct and social living. What standards, what rules and behaviour, will best secure the well-being of individuals, families, communities and nations? How are these standards to be promoted and enforced? The two approaches often use the same words as they debate these great questions – words like justice, rights, responsibility, duty, care, fairness – but the words do not always mean the same thing in the different discourses. Social work is at the sharp end of these debates, trying to help individuals and society.

This chapter introduces the core concepts that run throughout the book. It does so by highlighting four key pairings – rights and responsibilities, the individual and society, freedom and control, certainty and uncertainty. Later chapters add two more key pairings, reason and emotion (Chapter 4) and consensus and conflict (Chapter 5).

Box 1.1: Background: social work, law and ethics in the 1980s

The child protection scandals of the mid-1980s provide the background to the two fundamental questions in this book, about the relationship between law and ethics and the challenges of intervening the right way at the right time. There was a succession of high-profile cases where social workers were very heavily criticised for failing to prevent children being killed by their parents/carers. Two of the most prominent cases, attracting widespread media interest and public outrage, were those of Jasmine Beckford (Brent, 1985) and Kimberley Carlile (Greenwich, 1987).

The inquiries into these two cases were both chaired by a prominent lawyer of the time, Louis Blom-Cooper QC (also, incidentally, the co-editor of a book entitled *Law and Morality*, Blom-Cooper and Drewry, 1976). The reports are notable for their searing criticism of social workers for lacking knowledge of the law; for lacking understanding of the powers and responsibilities the law gave them; and for lacking readiness to exercise their statutory powers decisively and authoritatively. The report of the Jasmine Beckford inquiry argues that the legal context of social work is crucial:

We are strongly of the view that social work can, in fact, be defined *only* in terms of the functions required of its practitioners by their employing agency operating within a statutory framework.

(Brent, 1985: 12, emphasis original)

Then, just as these criticisms were at their height, came the Cleveland sexual abuse crisis (Cleveland is a county in north-east England). Between February and July 1987, two paediatricians in the area diagnosed 121 children as having been sexually abused. The cases were referred to the local authority social services department and over two-thirds of the children were separated from their parents or carers on an emergency basis (DHSS, 1988: 21, 172). Many of the parents criticised social workers for acting in hasty and authoritarian ways, assuming their guilt, not listening to them or the children, and making decisions without informing or consulting them (DHSS, 1988: 40–2). The affair became a national scandal, with social workers now being blamed for over-reacting. There was a public inquiry into the events, although it did not address the question of whether the children had really been abused. Instead, it concentrated on the procedural, managerial and legal issues (DHSS, 1988; and see Campbell, 1988 for a counterview to the official inquiry).

The Cleveland crisis became the catalyst for a major reform of child care legislation (although a range of other factors also lay behind the changes; see Eekelaar and Dingwall, 1990). The result was the Children Act 1989, which is still in force today. It introduced new concepts and legal orders for local authority social work to support families and protect children. It has been much amended over the years, but its key principles and provisions have endured. It did not solve the dilemmas of under-intervention and over-intervention, but gave a new framework for trying to strike the tricky balance between them. The fact that there continue to be child abuse deaths, despite all the legislation, all the publicity and all the procedures, shows just how difficult and uncertain the balances are.

The various inquiries in the 1980s set off an intense debate about the relationship between law and social work, and the proper place of the law in social work training (for example, Ball *et al.*, 1988; Stevenson, 1988; Braye and Preston-Shoot, 1990). The Beckford report, as we have seen, held that law is central to social work practice, its defining feature. Against this, one of the leading social work professors of the time, Olive Stevenson, argued that the pivot of social work is not law but an ethical duty of care to the client, and that it is 'dangerous and misleading to regard social work as a creation of law' (Stevenson, 1988: 44).

Blom-Cooper's view implies that if only social workers knew the law better, all would be well – social work is simply a matter of knowing and applying the law. It does not recognise that the law may have competing demands (e.g. to support families *and* to protect children), or that social workers may have additional principles and priorities, not just those specified in legislation. Stevenson's view is that ethics brings different and more demanding duties than just following the law. This independence is crucial, because social work must not be reduced to just doing what the government orders.

Braye and Preston-Shoot (1990: 343) argue that the two extreme positions both 'distort by over-simplification the reality of practice', which is that 'social workers sit uncomfortably between the two polarities'. They go on to say that 'the dilemmas posed by taking due account both of the law and the ethical duty of care in professional practice lead social workers into the eye of the storm' (1990: 335; for an up-dated picture, see Braye and Preston-Shoot, 2006). This fundamental tension is at the heart of this book.

Law and ethics: an uneasy marriage

The relationship between law and ethics can be seen as an uneasy marriage in which the partners rely heavily on each other, but sometimes misunderstand one another and often argue. There is a lifetime of mutual need *and* resentment, interdependence *and* tension. It might be a difficult relationship but it is a durable and dynamic one, always ready to adapt to new situations, but neither side willing to give way first. Like (some!) long-standing marriages, the two sides have a tendency to interrupt each other, and finish off each other's sentences (see Swain, 1989).

The roots of the ambivalence and creative tension can be summarised in terms of a number of key pairings. These are not independent, but overlap and interweave. They make for a complex and demanding environment. It is the context in which social work operates.

Rights and responsibilities

First, there are the tensions between rights and responsibilities. 'Rights' is a term with powerful legal and ethical meaning. There are 'human rights', as reflected in the United Nations' *Universal Declaration of Human Rights* (1948) and the *International Covenants on Human Rights* (1966). These treaties reflect the view that people have certain rights simply because they are human beings, independently of the laws of any particular nation. National laws and policies should protect and advance those rights.

It is usual to distinguish two broad types of human rights – civil and political rights ('first generation rights') such as the right to life, freedom from slavery, freedom from detention without due cause; and social, economic and cultural rights ('second generation rights') such as the right to an adequate standard of living, to health care and to education (see Ife, 2008).

Another way of categorising rights is to distinguish between negative and positive rights. Negative rights are 'freedoms *from* . . .' – for example, freedom from discrimination, or from undue interference by other individuals and the state. Positive rights are rights *to* something, such as fair pay, safe working conditions, a basic income. Sometimes it is a matter of which way you look at it – is it a freedom *from* unreasonable intervention, or a right *to* private life? It is both, because the negative rights do carry positive implications – for example, the right to freedom from inhuman treatment implies a positive duty on states to protect individuals from such treatment.

The European Convention on Human Rights contains first generation rights, 'freedoms from', but judgments from the European Court of Human Rights have developed the positive consequences – for example, positive duties on the state to protect children from inhuman and degrading treatment

Chapter 2

(Article 3 of the Convention). The European Convention was incorporated into UK law by the Human Rights Act 1998, and is of vital importance to social work and all public services in the UK. The rights in the Convention are outlined in Chapter 2, but discussed throughout the book.

Even if certain human rights are not upheld in the legislation and policy of a particular country, they can still carry powerful political and ethical force. For example, the right to freedom from inhuman treatment and the right to liberty can be used by campaigners to press for an end to torture and unwarranted detention, in all countries of the world. Furthermore, the language of rights is used by many groups to strengthen their claims to fairer treatment (or what they see as fairer treatment) –

Chapters 2 & 5

women's rights, disabled people's rights, prisoners' rights, fathers' rights and so on. So we can begin to understand human rights in terms of *freedom* and *fairness* (Equalities Review, 2007); but both these terms are controversial, as we shall see in later chapters, especially Chapter 2 on different dimensions of fairness, and Chapter 5 on different understandings of freedom.

In terms of the major ethical schools summarised in Chapter 4, human rights are often seen as a modern development of older, Kantian principles of categorical duties and of treating individuals as ends not means, respecting their dignity and worth as unique human beings. On the other hand, the notion that 'rights carry responsibilities' has become a well-used mantra in politics in the UK, reminding us that the rights of particular individuals and groups may have to balanced against the rights of the other members of society (e.g. MoJ, 2009a). So, certain individuals may claim a right to

Chapter 4

live in the UK, but, the politicians say, in that case they have to obey the laws of the land; or individuals may claim unemployment benefits, but in that case they have to be ready to take any work when it becomes available. This suggests a more utilitarian view of rights, with the overall good of society taking precedence (again, see Chapter 4).

A further aspect of the rights–responsibilities pairing is that if someone has got a right, then there is a question of whose responsibility it is to meet it; or at least, to ensure that there are no hindrances, so that it is possible for the person themselves to secure their entitlement if they so wish. This duty may fall in the first place on family members, or other citizens, but may become the responsibility of the state. It may be met through legal entitlements and protection, but also through the provision of public services, such as health, education, welfare benefits and social work. So we have to look at the responsibility of individuals *and* society in meeting people's rights, not just the responsibilities they carry themselves.

Individual and society

The second of the key pairings highlights the interactions between individual behaviour and duties, and the overall well-being of society. Law and ethics, in the western democratic tradition, are both concerned to strike the balance between the individual and society, regulating each side of the equation in order to preserve and advance the other. Both aim to regulate individual conduct in order to ensure the well-being of the community as a whole, but also to preserve individual freedoms against an over-bearing state or society.

But what comes first, the individual or society? For Kant, it is the individual. Kant's starting point is the notion of duty and the rational thinking of the autonomous individual. If this hypothetical person thinks through the issues sufficiently clearly, applying Kant's golden rule, the 'categorical imperative', they will know what they have to do, even if it is hard and they do not really want to do it. Doing one's duty prevails over the self-interest of the individual and even the apparent interests of others. Ultimately, society can only function well if everyone does their duty.

The utilitarians take a different angle. For them, the golden rule is 'the greatest good for the greatest number'. The interests of society prevail over the interests of the individual. Intriguingly, though, in order to achieve this, they rely on a particular view about the self-interests of individuals. For the traditional utilitarians, individuals are motivated not by reason but by a primary instinct to avoid pain and maximise pleasure, to gain the greatest happiness. The task of the legislator and the ethicist is to create a system of laws and values, rewards and sanctions that *uses* this primary instinct to ensure that people behave in the interests of society. In other words, desired behaviour is rewarded with pleasurable experiences such as praise, status, money; and undesired behaviour is punished by criticism, withdrawal of privileges, fines, imprisonment.

Individuals are shaped by the values of their society and the opportunities it brings them; but however powerful the social context, it is not all-encompassing. For a start, societies are diverse – they contain different groups, with different characteristics and interests. There are major differences of ethnicity, religion, age, gender and health, and people in these different groups may have different ideas about what constitutes 'the greatest good'. Things get even more complex when we realise that individuals belong to multiple social groupings (able-bodied white Polish female; physically disabled black British male, and so on), so may experience conflicting loyalties and demands within themselves. But this complexity and difference creates opportunities for change. It gives individuals the ideas and the space to *construct* their society, through their choices and their actions, perpetuating or challenging its norms and customs (Berger and Luckmann, 1967; Giddens, 1984).

Social work has a long interest in both sides of the individual–social tension. Payne (2006) argues that the distinctive feature of social work is its claim to achieve social change *through* work with individuals. But achieving this is not straightforward. Social workers can often help individuals to reach their goals, but sometimes they have to go against the wishes of the individual in the interests of others, and sometimes they have to refuse a service to an individual because resources are limited and the needs of others are considered greater (i.e. to maximise the greatest good).

There is a further aspect, that social workers themselves are individuals, members of particular social groupings and of larger society. So we have our individual backgrounds and abilities, beliefs and concerns; but how we practise is constrained by wider social values and priorities, by the law of the land, by the policies and resources of the organisations we work for, and by professional values and codes. Sometimes social workers can find themselves painfully caught between these different requirements.

Freedom and control

The third dimension focuses on the tensions between liberty and enforcement. Western societies place high value on individual autonomy, freedom from arbitrary interference by the state and the freedom to choose one's own way of life (discussed further in Chapter 5). However, as Bauman (1993) highlights, this is often a frightening prospect for those at the top of society. Will the lower orders really choose the right thing? So despite the widespread rhetoric of autonomy and choice, law and ethics both have a tendency to swing back towards authoritarianism and enforcement. The greatest challenge for society's leaders is to get people to think and behave in ways that they (the leaders) want them to. Ethics and law are ways to achieve this. Through education and moral advice, people can be taught

society's values; and if people believe that the rules are right, then it is much easier to enforce them. At the same time, legal methods can reinforce the moral lessons – as Bauman (1993: 9) puts it, 'the relentless pressure of legal sanctions [can] pour blood into the dry veins of philosophical argument'.

The most perfect form of control is when people do not even realise they are being controlled, when they are freely choosing to do their duty and comply with society's values, laws and policies (Foucault, 1977; Lukes, 2005). 'Free compliance' is the goal of education and socialisation, but taken too far it would leave us in a frightening, totalitarian society (as in George Orwell's *Nineteen Eighty-Four*: Orwell, 1949). To resist that, it is important to preserve, and value, the possibility of dissent and difference. So, freedom and control, rather than being simple opposites, are closely interwoven. They are both necessary, but there is always tension between them. Equally, law and ethics can complement one another in the processes of instilling and maintaining social values, but they never merge: there is always difference and tension between them (the obvious example is that some people might consider a certain law to be unethical).

The message about the interweaving of freedom and control has important implications for social work. Social workers have always been in the middle of this tension, trying to help people to take control of their own lives, but always having to be mindful of their powers and duties to exercise control over individuals, for their own safety or the safety of others. Sometimes social workers may use formal, legal measures to do so, such as taking a case to court, but more often they use informal techniques. This may start with counselling and advice, but can move through persuasion to threats of legal action, and even the withholding of services to get people to comply (e.g. Campbell and Davidson, 2009). It can be legally and ethically treacherous.

The ambiguities and dilemmas have been sharpened in recent years by the rise of 'personalisation' as a driving force for the reform of public services under the New Labour government of 1997–2010 (e.g. DH, 2008a), and continuing under the Conservative–Liberal Democrat coalition (e.g. DH, 2010a, b). The rhetoric is to give greater choice and control to service users, and social work is at the forefront of these developments, notably through the spread of direct payments and personal budgets. But there are critical voices that question how far this is truly motivated by the goals of empowerment and help, how much by mistrust and forcing people to take on more individual responsibilities, and how much by the lure of saving money (e.g. Ferguson, 2007; Scourfield, 2007). Questions also have to be asked about how to transfer control to service users whilst retaining responsibility for the well-being of individuals and society, and the fair use of limited resources. These debates come up throughout the book.

Certainty and uncertainty

The fourth pairing focuses on the tensions between the quest for certainty and the realities of ambiguity, complexity and change. We have already mentioned these ideas, but considering them as a separate pairing helps to draw out the lessons and challenges.

Ethical systems such as Kantianism and utilitarianism seek certainty in dealing with the difficult problems of life. Kantianism claims to bring certainty through the application of reason, to identify the right thing to do. Utilitarianism aims for certainty by calculating the happiness that a course of action will bring, and choosing the option that brings the greatest good to the greatest number. Both run up against the dilemmas and uncertainties of real life. The Kantians face uncertainty because in any particular situation there may be more than one reasonable course of action, or duties may point in different directions (for example, conflict between one's obligations as a parent and as an employee). The utilitarians face ambiguity because one can never fully predict all the consequences of one's decisions. Perhaps, in the long run, a different decision would have brought greater benefits?

Law also seeks certainty. It tries to remove uncertainty by reducing complex dilemmas to simple dichotomies – legal or illegal, guilty or not guilty, proven or not proven. This simplification serves law's objectives, to maintain social order. One way it tries to do this is by sending out messages that certain consequences will follow from certain actions, thus shaping people's expectations and behaviour. So, to take a simple example, it creates an expectation that driving too fast will lead to a fine and penalty points on one's driving licence, because that is what routinely happens to people who are caught for speeding. Repeated offences will lead to larger fines and more points, and eventually loss of the licence.

It may well be that most motorists get away with driving too fast on occasions, but nevertheless, law reinforces expectations about acceptable conduct through the punishments that it imposes on those who are caught.

To achieve this role in social control, law must send out simple and consistent messages. If it were otherwise, if it appeared arbitrary whether one got let off, a few penalty points or a lot, a light fine or a heavy one, there would be no reliable expectations and law would be ineffective. But like ethics, law runs up against the complex realities of life. Arguably, law has a limited impact on behaviour (how well

it really works in deterring offending is hotly contested, as discussed in Chapters 5 and 10), and no law can cover every eventuality. Laws have 'gaps', or perhaps circumstances change so that they become out of date. Lawyers are paid a lot of money to find the holes in the law, and to argue hard for alternative ways of interpreting and applying legislation. In reality, law is often neither clear nor consistent.

The cases that social workers deal with are more complex than the speeding example, and here the limitations and uncertainties often come to the fore. For example, what sort of contact should a parent be allowed with a child they have ill-treated? How far should a person be supported in their wishes, even though they place them at risk of harm? When should one deprive a person of their liberty in their own interests? Such difficulties and ambiguities are rife in social work, and legalistic approaches are, generally, not good at dealing with them (King and Trowell, 1992; Parton, 1998). Cases are complex and legislation can be ambiguous; that is why there is a hierarchy of courts, so that the hardest cases are decided by the most experienced judges. But in the end, after all the reports, all the appeals and all the arguing, cases come down to a basic either/or decision – guilty or not guilty, order or no order. This binary framework means that law's certainty can sometimes seem rather clumsy and unfair.

Having said that, there are times when social workers need to use the law to try to bring some control to uncertain and risky situations. Equally, there are times when families and individuals will use the law to try to resist social work intervention, or to get the sort of help that they want – in other words, to gain certainty from *their* point of view. So as with all the key pairings discussed in this chapter, the issues are not as simple as choosing one or the other, but seeing the value of both sides, recognising the benefits of certainty but also the importance of recognising ambiguity and valuing openness.

Conclusion

This chapter has introduced the key questions that guide this book, and four key pairings that show some of the complexities in the marriage of law and ethics, and the challenges they create for social work.

Legal and ethical approaches to human behaviour and the good society tend to look for certainty. The courts do so with their binary system of settling cases, legislators in the writing and passing of laws, policy makers in the regulations and procedures manuals that proliferate in social work. But we live in a world where uncertainty and complexity are the most common experiences, and social work is at the heart of such ambiguities. To remove the children, or to leave them at home? To enforce treatment on a person who is mentally unwell, or not? There are not often easy answers, but clear thinking about the legal and ethical dimensions can help us deal better with the questions. Social work's mixed and often contradictory functions, to work with individuals *and* for society, to empower *and* protect, make it an emblematic profession for an ambiguous world.

Questions for reflection

- Where do your personal values come from? Have your values changed in the course of your life? If so, what were the reasons?

- Think about Olive Stevenson's assertion that the pivot of social work is an ethical duty of care. What would you include in this duty? Make a list of the things you would include, and why they might be ambiguous or difficult to achieve. Are there any tensions with your personal values? It is more interesting to do this in a group, or to compare your answers with those of your colleagues. You may also find it useful to compare your answers with the ideas in the *Duty of Care Handbook* published by the public sector trade union, Unison (2011).

Useful websites and further reading

SCIE's e-learning resource on law and social work is a very useful introduction to legal principles in social work, and relevant law. It is an interactive site, with video and self-assessment activities. It is enjoyable and informative. www.scie.org.uk/publications/elearning/law/index.asp

There is a good range of textbooks about law for social workers. R. Johns (2011) *Using the Law in Social Work*, 5th edition, is a good introductory book.

The two leading overview books with all the essential law are:

- Brammer (2010) *Social Work Law*, 3rd edition.

- Brayne and Carr (2010) *Law for Social Workers*, 11th edition.

2 Fairness

This chapter discusses further key concepts for social work, law and ethics, namely justice, equality, human rights and care. These are terms that have great significance for all three, but do not always carry the same meaning in those different discourses. Indeed, all of them carry a variety of hotly contested meanings. At the heart of all of them are ideas about what is *fair* – notably, what amount of help, and what sort of help, is fair when people need extra care and support (fair for the individuals concerned and fair for society as a whole)? The challenge, of course, is that different people have very different ideas about what is fair, depending on their personal, professional, political and philosophical beliefs.

By way of introduction, it is possible to see two sides to each of justice, equality, human rights and care. For justice, there is an important distinction between formal justice and social justice. Formal justice relates to the courts, where (in theory) everyone is treated equally. Social justice is a broader concept that recognises deep-rooted inequalities in society, and calls for social and legal change to tackle them. In this sense, it is fair to offer special treatment to some people (positive action) to help redress the limited opportunities that they have had up until now (for example, favourable offers for students from poor families to take up university places). Likewise, equality has two aspects, equality of opportunity and treatment, and equality of outcome. Human rights can also be divided into two broad branches, as described in Chapter 1. Civil and political rights concern fair and equal treatment for people in the legal and political systems (e.g. the right to a fair hearing; 'one person, one vote') while social, economic and cultural rights underpin claims

Chapter 1

to special treatment for people who need extra help (e.g. the right to an adequate standard of living). Finally, the term 'duty of care' has very different meanings in legal and ethical contexts.

Justice

Justice in the courts, formal justice, is blind to differences between defendants – hence the statue of Justice, holding the sword and the scales, wears a blindfold. The decisions of the court are based on the legal provisions and the evidence, not favouritism or political bias (in theory). The same rules and procedures apply to everyone – that's fair. Having said that, the courts are not entirely blind to individual circumstances. There may be allowance for some individual characteristics – for example, younger offenders are treated differently to adults, those who committed their offence in very stressful situations may be given a lighter sentence. However, these are limited ways of adjusting the outcome for those individuals, they are not ways of changing society and creating better opportunities in the first place for those people and others like them.

Social justice, on the other hand, recognises that some people are disadvantaged by factors such as poverty or poor health, that certain groups of people suffer from discrimination and limited opportunities, and it aims to redress these imbalances. In this approach, justice does not mean treating everyone the same, but giving extra help to some, to bring them up to a more equal position. Social justice is not the aim of the courts unless there is a law about it, and the law has been broken. So, under the Equality Act 2010 it is illegal to discriminate against people with certain 'protected characteristics' (see further below). If someone considers that they have been discriminated against because of that characteristic, say, because they are gay, they could bring an action against the person who did so, and the case will be heard in court (or another relevant body, such as an employment tribunal). Note that the legal action has to be on grounds that are specific and covered by the law. A general complaint that homosexual people don't get the same opportunities as heterosexuals is not a matter for the courts. Grievances that are not covered by legislation would be a matter for pressure groups and political campaigns, and might then become law.

This takes us to the politics of justice, the public debates and arguments. In any particular situation, in the face of competing demands, what is the just thing to do? Answering this question involves far more than the law. It involves individual and social values, beliefs about rights and responsibilities, and about freedom and control. Amartya Sen gives a simple but effective example of the challenges in his book *The Idea of Justice* (2009), shown in Box 2.1

> ## Box 2.1: Anne, Bob or Carla? *The Idea of Justice* (Sen, 2009)
>
> Sen outlines the following scenario. You have to decide which of three children, Anne, Bob and Carla, should get a flute that they are quarrelling about (Sen, 2009: 13–15). Anne says that she should have it because she is the only one who can play it (the others agree this is true), and everyone will be happiest when they can enjoy listening to the beautiful music. Bob claims it because he is the poorest, and the only one who has no toys of his own (the other two accept this). He will enjoy it the most by far, because the others already have more than enough. Carla claims it because she made it. She spent months working on it without any help from the others (they acknowledge this), but now they say they want it.
>
> • What is your decision? What are your reasons?
>
> • Discuss the scenario with your fellow students. What do you agree or disagree about?
>
> • What parallels with social work do you see, or messages for social work?

Justice as fairness

John Rawls' famous book, *A Theory of Justice* (revised edition 1999, first edition 1971) sets out his approach of 'justice as fairness'. It has become a well-known starting point for debates about social justice. Rawls' objective is to balance social justice with individual freedom and difference. Rawls' argument is that the most just society will be governed by two basic principles:

• that each person should have equal rights to the greatest possible degree of individual liberty, compatible with the same degree of freedom for others;

• that social and economic inequalities are allowed, but (a) only in so far as they bring benefits for everyone, in particular the greatest benefit to the least advantaged; and (b) there must be equality of opportunity.

To illustrate his argument, Rawls describes a hypothetical situation in which people are designing their future society from scratch. He calls this 'the original position'. All the participants are rational and free, and all have equal rights in the debate (this is the basis on which he considers his model 'fair'). The vital point is that the participants do not know what their own position in the future society will be. They have to decide on the arrangements behind a 'veil of ignorance'. In these circumstances, how big a gap between the rich and the poor would they allow? Between the opportunities for men and women, black people and white people, disabled people and able-bodied people? Between those who work hard and those who choose not to? Remember, when the veil is drawn back they might be one of the people with limited skills, with unconventional views, with bad luck, or who belongs to an unfavoured group.

Rawls argues that people in the original position would choose those two principles of justice as the basis for their new society. The implication, of course, is that we should act according to those principles in our own society.

Rawls discusses his theory of justice in relation to the dominant western ethical approaches of utilitarianism and Kantianism (see Chapter 4). His model allows inequality insofar as it serves the well-being of society, but he distinguishes his position from utilitarianism because of his emphasis on individual rights and the well-being of the least advantaged. Rawls regards his theory as a duty-based theory in the tradition of Immanuel Kant. He considers the original position to be an interpretation of Kant's arguments that moral principles have to be universal and a matter of rational choice, made by free and equal rational beings (Rawls, 1999: 221–5).

One difficulty, as Sen's example of Anne, Bob and Carla shows so well, is that free and equal rational beings can give different answers about the right thing to do. There is a good case for each of the children to have the flute. Sen argues that a theory of justice has to allow for a plurality of views and continuing disagreements. Having said that, he is not a relativist, and believes that some decisions are more just than others. Good arguments should prevail over poor ones. The key steps are to discuss the issues openly, to try to reach agreement through public reasoning; and to act pragmatically, tackling the worst injustices first, making the world a bit more just, a step at a time.

Equality

Treating all people fairly, not discriminating against people, valuing difference and challenging oppression and inequality are fundamental social work values (e.g. IFSW and IASSW, 2004; BASW, 2012; Dominelli, 2002, 2009; Thompson, 2011). It is usual to think of two faces of equality – equality of opportunity or treatment, and equality of outcome. Rawls' model of justice includes equality of opportunity, but not outcome. But the relationship between these two aspects is more blurred than this allows – genuinely equal opportunites are likely to result in more equal outcomes, less inequality of wealth and health; and in turn, outcomes determine further opportunities. The report of the National Equality Panel (2010) gives an up-to-date picture of levels of inequality in the United Kingdom, highlighting the powerful, long-term impact of economic advantage and disadvantage across people's lives and their children's lives. It concludes that equality of opportunity is very hard to achieve 'when there are such wide differences in the resources which people and their families have to help them develop their talents and fulfil their diverse potentials' (National Equality Panel, 2010: 36).

The law on equality in England, Wales and Scotland has been up-dated by the Equality Act 2010. This was passed by the Labour government before it lost the 2010 general election. The purpose was to consolidate and strengthen the wide range of anti-discrimination and equal opportunities legislation. The result is a large act, with 218 sections and 28 schedules. Most of it came into force in October 2010, under the coalition government.

There is a long history of legislation against discrimination on the grounds of race, sex and disability, and more recently age, religion and belief, and sexual orientation. The Act brings these and other aspects together by specifying nine 'protected characteristics'. Discriminating against a person (that is, treating them less favourably than another, directly or indirectly), harassment and victimisation on the basis of any of these characteristics is illegal. The nine characteristics are listed in s. 4 of the Act:

- age;

- disability;

- gender reassignment;

- marriage and civil partnership;

- pregnancy and maternity;

- race;

- religion or belief;

- sex;

- sexual orientation.

Furthermore, there are positive duties on public authorities to promote equality of opportunity (i.e. more than simply not discriminating). This is s. 149 of the Act, the public sector equality duty, which came into force in April 2011. It applies to eight of the protected characteristics, the exclusion being marital and civil partnership (note: *discrimination* on the basis of marital or civil partnership status is illegal, but public authorities do not have a duty to *promote* any position on them). Positive action is allowed to help people overcome the effects of disadvantage connected to the protected characteristics (s. 158), and 'reasonable adjustments' for disabled people must be made where possible (s. 20).

Section 1 of the Act was going to introduce a new duty on public authorities to promote equality of outcome for people suffering from 'socio-economic disadvantage' (that is, disadvantages linked to social class and poverty). This would have been a general duty, to be borne in mind at the level of policy-making and strategic decisions, not a specific duty owed to individuals. The coalition government declared that it would not implement this part of the Act, claiming that it would create more bureaucracy, not achieve greater equality (HM Government, 2010a: 8).

The lead government body for implementing the Act is the Government Equalities Office (GEO). This is part of the Home Office, but works across all government departments. It also takes the lead on implementing the coalition government's *Equality Strategy* (HM Government, 2010a). The Strategy emphasises the two goals of building a strong economy and a fairer society, and two 'principles of equality' – equality of opportunity and equality of treatment (note, not equality of outcome). The report of the National Equality Panel (2010) is now in the archived section of the GEO website.

The new Strategy makes a number of challenging points about the relationship between legislation and social change. It gives a number of examples, which (it says) show the limitations of the law. It observes that despite years of equalities legislation, women are still paid significantly less than men, there are large differences in employment rates for people from different racial and ethnic groups, and people with disabilities are still victims of bullying and hate crimes. The Strategy makes a similar point about public spending – despite large amounts of money being spent on equality of opportunity, there are still substantial differences in areas such as academic achievement of children from poorer and wealthier families, and life expectancy of richer and poorer people (HM Government, 2010a: 8).

Another crucial body is the Equality and Human Rights Commission (EHRC). One of its roles is to protect, enforce and promote equality across the nine protected characteristics. It has produced a number of statutory codes of practice to go with the Act (e.g. on equal pay, employment and public services), and also a series of non-statutory guides (for employers, workers, service providers, service users, education providers and public sector bodies). It argues for greater social justice, a society 'where every individual has the opportunity to achieve their potential, and people treat each other with dignity and respect' (EHRC, 2010: 12).

Human rights

The Human Rights Act 1998 (HRA 1998) incorporated the European Convention on Human Rights (ECHR) into UK law. It came into force in October 2000. It has had, and continues to have, a major impact on UK law generally, all public services, and social work policy and practice (e.g. McDonald, 2007). The rights in the Convention are summarised in Box 2.2. They are first generation, civil and political rights, mainly expressed in terms of freedom from undue state interference, but in Chapter 1 we have already noted that negative rights can translate into positive duties on the state to secure

Chapters 1 & 3

them. However, it is important to notice that there are very few absolute rights. Most are limited or qualified. Article 3 is an absolute right, with no allowance for any exceptions. Articles 2, 4(2) and 5 are examples of limited rights, which can be overruled under certain conditions specified in the article itself. Qualified rights (8, 9, 10 and 11) can only be infringed on grounds that are legal, necessary and proportionate (see further in Chapter 3).

Box 2.2: Key articles from the European Convention on Human Rights

Art. 2: Right to life

1   Everyone's right to life shall be protected by law. No one shall be deprived of his life intentionally save in the execution of a sentence of a court.

Art. 3: Prohibition of torture

1   No one shall be subjected to torture or to inhuman or degrading treatment or punishment.

Art. 4: Freedom from slavery and forced labour

1   No one shall be held in slavery or servitude.

2   No one shall be required to perform forced or compulsory labour.

Note: Work done as part of a court sentence or military service is not included.

Art. 5: Right to liberty and security

1   Everyone has the right to liberty and security of person.

Note: Lawful arrest and detention of persons convicted or suspected of committing a crime is allowed, as is lawful detention of persons of 'unsound mind'.

Art. 6: Right to a fair trial

1   In the determination of his civil rights and obligations or of any criminal charge against him, everyone is entitled to a fair and public hearing within a reasonable time by an independent and impartial tribunal established by law. Judgment shall be pronounced publicly but the press and public may be excluded from all or part of the trial in the interest of morals, public order or national security in a democratic society, where the interests of juveniles or the protection of the private life of the parties so require.

Note: The text refers to a hearing not just a trial, and covers the decisions of administrative bodies, not just courts. Many sorts of social work meetings and panels will be included, in so far as they affect people's rights under the ECHR (for example, child protection case conferences). This does not mean they have to comply with every aspect of Article 6 (e.g. to be held in public) but there must be a right of appeal to a body that does (DCA, 2006a). The principles of a fair hearing and fair decision-making certainly apply.

Art. 8: Right to respect for private and family life

1   Everyone has the right to respect for his private and family life, his home and his correspondence.

2   There shall be no interference by a public authority with the exercise of this right except such as is in accordance with the law and is necessary in a democratic society in the

interests of national security, public safety or the economic well-being of the country, for the prevention of disorder or crime, for the protection of health or morals, or for the protection of the rights and freedoms of others.

Art. 9: Freedom of thought, conscience and religion

1. Everyone has the right to freedom of thought, conscience and religion; this right includes freedom . . . to manifest his religion or belief, in worship, teaching, practice and observance.

Note: This is a qualified right, along the lines outlined for Article 8.

Art. 10: Freedom of expression

1 Everyone has the right to freedom of expression. This right shall include freedom to hold opinions and to receive and impart information and ideas without interference by public authority and regardless of frontiers.

Note: This is a qualified right, along the lines outlined for Article 8.

Art. 11: Freedom of assembly and association

1 Everyone has the right to freedom of peaceful assembly and to freedom of association with others, including the right to form and to join trade unions for the protection of his interests.

Note: this is a qualified right, along the lines outlined for Article 8.

Art. 12: Right to marry and found a family

1 Men and women of marriageable age have the right to marry and to found a family, according to the national laws governing the exercise of this right.

Art. 14: Prohibition of discrimination

1 The enjoyment of the rights and freedoms set forth in this Convention shall be secured without discrimination on any ground such as sex, race, colour, language, religion, political or other opinion, national or social origin, association with a national minority, property, birth or other status.

Note: This is not a right to freedom from discrimination in all aspects of life, but only applies to the other rights listed in the ECHR.

> As well as the main body of the Convention, there are a number of additional protocols, for example:
>
> **Protocol 1, Art. 2: Right to education**
>
> No person shall be denied the right to education ... the state shall respect the right of parents to ensure that such education and teaching is in conformity with their religious and philosophical convictions.
>
> Note: The UK entered a reservation to this article. It accepts the principle of education in conformity with parents' convictions, but only so far as it is compatible with the efficient provision of education and reasonable public expenditure.

The implementation of the HRA 1998 enables UK citizens to take action in the UK courts on matters covered by the ECHR. Furthermore, the Act makes it illegal for any public body to act in any way that is incompatible with a convention right (s. 6, HRA 1998). The term 'public body' includes (amongst others) central government departments, local authorities, the police and the courts. Section 3 of the Act requires courts to interpret and apply UK legislation in such a way that it is compatible with the ECHR. If this is not possible, then the courts may issue a declaration of incompatibility and the government will have to consider amending the legislation.

The Convention has proved controversial, with some people resenting European interference and arguing that it allows criminals to get away with their crimes. In 2006, the Labour government published a review of the implementation of the Human Rights Act (DCA, 2006b), which defended it. Even so, Labour was at pains to assert the importance of people having responsibilities, not just rights, and to that end proposed a new UK Bill of Rights and Responsibilities (MoJ, 2009a). There are a number of useful publications which show the value of the Convention and argue against the myths and misunderstandings about it (e.g. DCA, 2006a, b; BIHR, 2008; EHRC, 2008, 2009). Bingham (2010: 84) challenges the critics with two provocative questions: which of the rights in the Convention would you discard? And would you rather live in a country in which these rights were not protected?

Disputes arise regularly about the powers of the European Court to overturn UK law, policy and court decisions. A leading example is the European Court ruling that it is illegal for the UK to have a blanket ban on all convicted prisoners to stop them voting (*Hirst v United Kingdom (No. 2)* [2005]). The UK had delayed responding to this judgment, but the issue became prominent again in 2010, with the Prime Minister, David Cameron, saying that the thought of giving prisoners the vote made him 'physically ill'. In March 2011, the government set up an independent commission on a new UK bill of rights, which is due to report by the end of 2012.

Duty of care

As noted in Chapter 1 (Box 1.1), it has been held that the heart of social work is an ethical duty of care. However, the term 'duty of care' also has a distinctive legal meaning, and there are important differences between the two. It might seem obvious that a social worker owes a duty of care to everyone with whom they work (e.g. Unison, 2011). They may do in an ethical sense, but in a legal sense it is not at all straightforward. Under English common law, the duty of care is concerned with not doing harm, rather than a positive obligation to do good; but also, it excludes certain sorts of harm and certain sorts of relationship from the duty of care. It *limits* the circumstances under which a person who has been harmed by the actions or inactions of another may be able to sue the other person for damages in negligence (compensation).

It may be surprising to know, but until relatively recently the courts held that social workers did not have a common law duty of care to children in child protection investigations. This is because one of the grounds for imposing a common law duty of care is that it is 'fair, just and reasonable' to do so. In the case of *X (Minors) v Bedfordshire County Council* [1995], the House of Lords held that it was not.

This was a case where four children claimed damages against the local authority for not protecting them from physical and psychological harm from their parents. The local authority had first known about the case in October 1987, but did not remove the children until April 1992, during which time they continued to suffer severe ill-treatment and neglect. The House of Lords held that there was no duty of care for a number of reasons to do with wider public policy, rather than the specific facts of the case.

The main factors included that local authority social workers do not make decisions by themselves, but in conjunction with other agencies, so it is unfair to punish one agency; and that the decisions are very difficult, requiring delicate balancing of rights and priorities, and it would not be fair, once one has the benefit of hindsight, to blame workers for honest mistakes. Also, if local authorities were always worried about being sued, this would make them unduly cautious, afraid to make decisions that carried any risk; and furthermore, the costs of paying damages would reduce the money available for front-line services.

At that time, the Human Rights Act 1998 had not been passed and the European Convention was not part of UK law, so the children's lawyers could not take action under it in the UK courts. However, having used all the domestic options, they could then take the case to the European Court of Human Rights. Here it was known as *Z v United Kingdom* [2001]. The European Court held that there had been a breach of the children's right to freedom from inhuman and degrading treatment (Article 3). It awarded compensation to the children (see Miles, 2001; Bailey-Harris and Harris, 2002).

The passing of the Human Rights Act 1998 is having an on-going impact on the courts' approach to the duty of care. The position now is that when investigating allegations of child abuse, public authorities do have a common law duty of care towards the children, but not towards the parents.

That was the decision of the House of Lords in the case of *D v East Berkshire Community Health NHS Trust* [2005], upholding an earlier decision in the Court of Appeal. The case involved three separate appeals. In each case, the child concerned had been separated from their parents because of suspicions of child abuse. Subsequently it became clear that the children had not been abused, and they were returned home. The parents claimed for psychiatric harm caused to them by the false accusations or their consequences.

On a majority of 4–1, the law lords held that there was no duty of care to the parents. The majority reasoning was that if a social worker or doctor had to be mindful of the likelihood of being sued by the parents, this might inhibit them from investigating matters thoroughly. The primary patient, or service user, is the child, and their safety has to come first. That is not to say that the parents' interests should be disregarded, and workers still have to act in good faith, not recklessly. If an individual's practice departs significantly from what a reasonable professional would be expected to do, there may be grounds for a claim in negligence (*W and Others v Essex CC and Another* [2000]); otherwise, poor practice can be pursued through complaint procedures or other legal channels. Also, the legal limitations on the duty of care do not protect social workers or their agencies from public and media criticism when things go wrong; and no doubt the individuals concerned would feel terrible about what had happened. It is likely they would be held to account, or at least hold themselves to account, against professional and ethical standards, even if protected from legal action under the law of negligence.

So, the legal duty of care sends out a message about how people should treat one another, exercising due care. But we can see that it is not only about imposing responsibilities on individuals or public bodies, telling them how they should behave. It is also about limiting the circumstances in which people can make a claim. Not every relationship carries a legal duty of care, so not every harm entitles the victim to damages in negligence. Another example of this is given in Box 2.3.

Box 2.3: Duty of care: *X and Y v London Borough of Hounslow* **[2009]**

This case concerned a couple with learning disabilities who lived with their two children in a council flat. In summer 2000 they were befriended by a group of local youths who began exploiting the couple, using their flat for drug taking, underage sex and storing stolen goods. On occasions they were threatening and abusive towards the couple. The social worker had reported this several times to the housing department, calling on them to make the family a higher priority for re-housing (they already had a long-standing application for re-housing). Before anything was done, in November 2000, the youths effectively imprisoned the family in their own flat for a weekend and put them through a truly awful ordeal of assaults and abuse.

Three young men were convicted of the assaults and given custodial sentences. The couple took action against the local authority for negligence, arguing that they knew about the risk but had failed to protect them. The case reached the High Court in 2008, which upheld their claim, saying that the local authority did owe them a common law duty of care, and had breached it by failing to move them even though they knew about the danger. The couple were awarded damages of £97,000. Hounslow denied liability and appealed against the decision.

The case went to the Court of Appeal later in 2008, which overturned the decision (the judgment was delivered on 2 April 2009). It upheld the council's argument that it did not have a common law duty of care to protect adults with learning disabilities from attacks by third parties; and what is more, even if they had, they had not breached it because they had not acted negligently (paras 10, 65, 90, 95). There was no duty of care to re-house the couple, even though the authority knew about the risks. This was because it had fulfilled its statutory responsibilities about re-housing them, and it would not be 'fair, just or reasonable' to impose any extra duty, bearing in mind that the authority had to balance the couple's circumstances against those of other deserving cases and the rights of other tenants. As regards the adult social care department, it also was fulfilling its statutory duties, and these did not give rise to a common law duty of care without something extra, such as the council assuming responsibility to protect the couple from harm by third parties. This it had not done. They were adults living independent lives in the community, vulnerable though they were, and life has its risks. Further, the social worker's approach was one that a reasonable social worker could reasonably take and, indeed, she 'behaved impeccably throughout' (para. 95). No-one could have reasonably foreseen the awful events of that weekend.

Subsequently, the couple and X's mother applied to the European Court of Human Rights (*X, Y and Z v the United Kingdom* [2011]). Their main claims were that the local authority had failed to protect them from inhuman and degrading treatment (Article 3), and had allowed a violation of their private and family life (Article 8). The family and the UK government reached a 'friendly settlement' in July 2011. The family agreed to drop the case in return for payments totalling around £60,000.

Conclusion

The international definition of social work produced by the International Federation of Social Workers and the International Association of Schools of Social Work, asserts that 'Principles of human rights and social justice are fundamental to social work' (IFSW and IASSW, 2001), but this chapter has highlighted some of the complexities and controversies that lie behind such phrases. There are different dimensions to core concepts such as justice, human rights, equality and care. Striking the balance between them is a challenge in the day-to-day practice of individual social workers, but also goes way beyond that, involving law and politics. This is an important message in this book, to always try to set individual practice in context.

The next chapter adds to the picture by describing the legal system in England and Wales, and the key legal principles for trying to strike the balances in policy and in particular cases.

Questions for reflection

- Do you think the coalition government was right or wrong in deciding not to implement s. 1 of the Equality Act 2010? What are your reasons for your answer?

- There is no doubt that inequality and discrimination persist despite much legislation and public spending. What do you think the reasons are for this, and what should be done? What understandings of justice, equality and human rights do your answers reflect?

- Do you think prisoners should be allowed to vote? List your reasons, and discuss the question with your colleagues.

- What do you think about the decision in *X and Y v London Borough of Hounslow*?

Useful websites and further reading

Equality and Human Rights Commission: www.equalityhumanrights.com

Government Equalities Office: www.homeoffice.gov.uk/equalities/equality-government/

UK Human Rights blog: www.ukhumanrightsblog.com

Ife (2008) *Human Rights and Social Work: Towards Rights-Based Practice.*

Craig, Burchardt and Gordon (eds) (2008) *Social Justice and Public Policy: Seeking Fairness in Diverse Societies.*

Dorling (2010) *Injustice: Why Social Inequality Persists.*

3 The legal framework

This chapter introduces the legal framework for social work in England. The purpose is to give an overview of the major structures and principles as they relate to social work policy and practice. The governmental systems are different in Wales, Scotland and Northern Ireland (the Welsh Assembly Government, the Scottish Parliament and the Northern Ireland Assembly), but subject to the overall sovereignty of the UK Parliament in London. The judicial system is the same for England and Wales ('English law'), but different in Scotland and Northern Ireland; but the highest court of appeal for all the systems (except Scottish criminal law) is the UK Supreme Court in London. Despite the differences, the key distinctions to be discussed in this chapter are essential in all the countries. These are the differences between statute law and case law, and the European dimensions of each; law and guidance; criminal law and civil law; and powers and duties. The chapter also considers the principles of lawful decision-making by public authorities.

English law is made by Parliament and by the courts, and by the European Union (directly or indirectly), and under the influence of the European Court of Human Rights. The different elements interweave, sometimes reinforcing and sometimes challenging one another. We shall say more about each of them in turn. The starting point is the distinction between statute law and case law. Statute law is the term used for Acts of Parliament, the law created by politicians and civil servants rather than judges. Case law is the law created by the courts, as they decide cases and interpret the statutes, applying them to the facts of the case.

Politics and statute law

It is important to remember that Acts of Parliament are political products, not simply legal documents. They are passed and implemented by the government of the time, reflecting the public issues of the day, the amount of money available to fund services, the government's political priorities and their interpretation of 'social justice' (for example, whether social justice is better served if taxpayers or students themselves pay for university courses).

The process for making law in Parliament often starts with the government publishing a 'green paper' or a 'white paper', outlining the problem and possible solutions. Even before them, there will usually have been considerable discussions and lobbying from professional or special interest groups to change the law. A green paper is an early stage in the process, and may not always be used. It usually leads to further consultation with members of the public and the relevant organisations. If the government decides to take the matter forward, there will then be a white paper, which contains more specific proposals. After that, there are further consultations, possibly including the publication of a draft bill. If the government decides to proceed there will then be a bill, which is the proposed legislation. The bill goes through a number of stages, usually starting in the House of Commons before going to the House of Lords and then back to the Commons. The bill is debated in each House, and goes to a committee stage in each House. This involves a smaller group of politicians with a special interest in the topic, making a detailed study of each clause of the bill (n.b. bills have clauses, acts have sections). It is likely that the bill will be amended during these deliberations. The House of Lords can amend a bill and can delay it, but cannot refuse a bill that has been passed by the House of Commons. As the government has the majority of seats in the Commons, it should always be able to get bills passed as it wishes, eventually, unless there is a rebellion by its own MPs. The threat of rebellion means that unpopular legislation can involve a lot of political bargaining and arm-twisting. The parliamentary process can be completed very quickly for bills that are a government priority, but can take up to a year or more.

Eventually the bill receives Royal Assent and becomes an Act. It might come into force straightaway, but more likely there will be further delay before it is implemented, to allow for necessary arrangements to be made. This could include the publication of regulations and guidance to accompany the Act.

A feature of the political process is that new Acts can be passed to deal with new problems, public issues or political priorities. These may simply replace the old law, but just as likely they will repeal parts of it whilst retaining others, or add new requirements on top of the existing law, or amend it in places. This can lead to some very complicated situations, where a number of different Acts with different terms and provisions address the same or related topics. The law on adult social care in England has become a prime example of this. In 2008 the Law Commission described it as 'inadequate, often incomprehensible and outdated' (Law Commission, 2008: 10). The Law Commission undertook a review and produced its final report in 2011, with proposals to reform and simplify the law on adult social care (see Law Commission, 2010, 2011; House of Commons Health Committee, 2012). A White Paper was due to be published in summer 2012.

Legislation and guidance

Acts of Parliament are known as primary legislation. In order to bring them into effect, it is often necessary for the government to pass many more detailed *regulations*. These are known as 'delegated legislation', or 'secondary legislation', and usually take the form of 'statutory instruments'. They are just as much law as primary legislation. In child and family social work a prominent example is the *Care Planning, Placement and Case Review Regulations 2010* (which came into force on 1 April 2011: HM Government, 2010b).

The government may also issue *directions* to local authorities, if the primary legislation permits them to do so. Such directions have the force of law and must be followed. An example from adult social care is the *Community Care Assessment Directions 2004*, issued under s. 47(4) of the National Assistance Act 1948.

The relevant government department may also issue *guidance* to the agencies and professionals who have to implement the law. Often this guidance is issued by the government as 'statutory guidance', also known as 'policy guidance'. Statutory guidance to local authorities on social care is usually issued under s. 7 of the Local Authority Social Services Act (LASSA) 1970. Although it is not law in the same way as the primary and secondary legislation, it must be followed unless there are good reasons to deviate from it, and even then authorities cannot take a substantially different course (*R v Islington London Borough Council, ex parte Rixon* [1997]). The courts will normally expect local authorities to have followed statutory guidance, so there must be strong and clearly recorded reasons for not doing so.

Examples of statutory guidance are the eligibility criteria for adult social care, *Prioritising Need in the Context of Putting People First* (DH, 2010b), and Part 1 of the *Working Together* guidance for safe-guarding children from neglect and abuse (HM Government, 2010c). (A new version of the *Working Together* guidance was due to be published in 2012.)

The government may also publish 'practice guidance', which sets out what the relevant department holds to be good practice. Local authorities are required to 'have regard' to this. There is an expectation that it will be followed, but it is another notch down again, so there is more leeway to take a different course of action. As always though, there must be well-argued and clearly recorded reasons for the course of action. Part 2 of the 2010 *Working Together* guidance is classed as practice guidance.

Some legislation allows the government to publish 'codes of practice'. Again, these do not have the full force of law, but failure to follow them could have serious implications for the agency or individual worker. Different codes have different requirements, but an example is the Mental Health Act 1983 Code of Practice, revised in 2008 (DH, 2008b). It is discussed further in Chapter 11. Section 118 of the Mental Health Act specifies certain categories of people who are required to 'have regard' to it. Failure to follow the code could lead to disciplinary action, and might be a basis for legal challenge (e.g. judicial review).

Courts and case law

Case law operates on the principle of *precedent*. This is that courts should follow the decisions made in previous cases by superior courts – these take precedence. This way, a common law evolves that applies across all the country and to all similar cases. Having said that, a judge may well decide that the facts of a particular case are different from previous cases, and so they are not strictly bound by previous judgments. In child care cases, for example, it is not unusual for judges to observe that every case is unique and has to be decided in the light of the specific circumstances and best interests of the individual child. Even so, they have to be mindful of the statutory requirements and the general judicial principles that shape the way other cases have been decided. So usually common law and statutory law are complementary; but if there is a clash, statute law prevails. The courts cannot overturn an Act of Parliament, however much they may dislike it (but they can overturn regulations). However, they do interpret and apply the law, and may do so in ways that the politicians did not quite intend. If that happens Parliament might amend the legislation to remove the ambiguity.

The court system works as a hierarchy, and is split between the civil courts and the criminal courts (see below for an outline of the differences between criminal and civil law). It is also important to remember the role of the various *tribunals* that deal with specialist areas of the law, such as employment, immigration, social security, mental health, and care standards. Most tribunals that deal with appeals against decisions of public bodies were reorganised into a two-tier system in November 2008, as a result of the Tribunals, Courts and Enforcement Act 2007. There is a generic First-tier Tribunal, which is sub-divided into specialist areas, and an Upper Tribunal that hears appeals from them.

1   At the bottom level of the court system are the magistrates' courts, which deal with most cases (adult criminal matters, youth offending, family proceedings and care proceedings under the Children Act 1989).

2   The next level up has the Crown Court, dealing with the more serious criminal cases and appeals from the magistrates' court; and the county court, which deals with civil matters including divorce and more complex family or care proceedings.

3   Above that comes the High Court, dealing with more complex cases again and appeals from the lower courts. It is split into three divisions. The *Family Division* deals with family matters, child care cases and adoption. The *Chancery Division* deals with financial matters such as bankruptcy and probate. The *Queen's Bench Division* deals with a wide range of matters. It includes the Administrative Court, which deals with judicial review (see below). There is also the Court of Protection, which deals with matters where people lack mental capacity to make decisions. This was established as a separate court at High Court level by the Mental Capacity Act 2005, and came into being in October 2007 (see Chapter 7).

Chapter 7

4   Above the High Court comes the Court of Appeal, with criminal and civil divisions.

5   Beyond that, at the top of the domestic system, comes the Supreme Court. This was established in October 2009, and took over from the House of Lords as the highest UK court, hearing appeals on cases of the greatest public importance. But even the Supreme Court has to take account of European Union legislation and judgments from the European Court of Human Rights. Most of the cases that the Supreme Court hears turn on the interpretation and application of the European Convention on Human Rights.

Two European dimensions

European integration means that there are now two new dimensions to the old distinction between statute law and case law. The European Union (EU) passes laws that apply to the United Kingdom, and can be enforced by the European Court of Justice. The European Court of Human Rights (ECtHR), delivers judgments on cases that have to be taken into account by courts and public authorities in the United Kingdom. It is important to be clear that these two European dimensions are separate bodies of law, and separate courts.

The European Union

The EU is an association of (currently) 27 nations, with a European Parliament that passes legislation which all member countries must uphold. EU legislation comes in the form of treaties, regulations and directives, mainly to do with economic and trade matters, but often with a human and social rights aspect. Regulations apply directly in member states, as if they were national law, whereas directives require the countries to develop their own legislation to achieve the objectives. As examples, there is an EU regulation on the rights of disabled people when travelling by air (Regulation 1107/2006/EC) and a directive on data protection (Directive 95/46/EC) which led the UK government to pass the Data Protection Act 1998 (see Chapter 12).

National parliaments cannot pass laws which do not comply with EU law. Member states which do not comply may be taken to the European Court of Justice, in Luxembourg. The decisions of the Court of Justice are binding on all UK courts.

The European Court of Human Rights

The European Court of Human Rights (ECtHR) is part of the Council of Europe, a body of (currently) 47 nations. It is based in Strasbourg, France. States that belong to the Council of Europe agree to be bound by the European Convention on Human Rights (ECHR), which was discussed in Chapter 2.

Chapter 2

Individuals who consider that their rights under the Convention have been infringed may take action against their state for committing or not preventing this. It is not possible under the ECHR to take action against individuals, or private and voluntary organisations. Action may be taken in their own national courts, if the Convention has been incorporated into their national law, or in the ECtHR itself. European human rights law is binding on all member nations, but there is some leeway for inter-pretation to take account of different national circumstances, known as the 'margin of appreciation'. Furthermore, the ECtHR does not have as tight a notion of precedent as the English system, regarding the Convention as a 'living instrument', so the interpretation of the Convention can change.

Criminal law and civil law

Another key legal distinction is between criminal law and civil law. Criminal law covers matters such as murder, robbery and drunk driving, where the consequences of the action are not only harmful to individual victims and their families, but harmful to all society. They threaten the peacefulness and order of society, so everyone has an interest in preventing them, and therefore usually the state takes the action against accused person. So, cases in the criminal courts are generally led by the Crown Prosecution Service, with the state as prosecutor and the accused person as the defendant. Given that some criminal offences can lead to a person being sent to prison, in some cases for life, the court has to be satisfied that the person is guilty *beyond reasonable doubt*.

Civil law cases, on the other hand, are between individuals or organisations. Examples are divorce, disputes about employment or business contracts, or claims for compensation because of an accident. Civil law can be further divided to public and private matters: when the organisation involved is a public body, such as a local authority, it is a matter of public law.

The state has an interest in ensuring that civil matters are resolved effectively, to maintain a peaceful and orderly society, so it provides the legal framework to resolve them (laws and courts). However, the case is not taken to court by the state, but by one of the parties. The party bringing the case is referred to as the applicant or claimant, and the other side as the defendant or respondent. The outcomes may be an order to settle the matter (e.g. a divorce), an award of compensation or an injunction to stop the behaviour that has caused the problem. Failure to obey a civil order may be a criminal matter. Decisions in the civil courts are made on the *balance of probabilities*.

Child care proceedings are a striking example of a public law matter, dealt with in the civil courts, where the issues and consequences are of profound personal significance and social importance. To remove someone's child from them against their wishes is surely as extreme an intervention by the state as any term of imprisonment, yet these cases are decided on the balance of probabilities, not beyond reasonable doubt. Whether there should be a higher standard of proof in care proceedings because of their serious consequences is a question that has come up in court judgments, but the case of *Re B* [2008] has clarified that the test is the ordinary civil one, the balance of probabilities ('more likely than not'). The point is that the purpose of care proceedings is to protect the child, not to prosecute the parents. No-one is found guilty in care proceedings, although no doubt it feels like this to many of the parents. Sometimes there are 'findings of fact' against a parent, that on the civil test the court considers he or she did abuse the child; but the law does not require anyone to be blamed in care proceedings. A parent with learning disabilities, for example, may not be able to provide the required level of care, but no-one would want to blame them for that. Indeed, most parents in care proceedings do not mean to harm their children, but their own problems and vulnerabilities limit what they can offer.

Powers and duties

A further key distinction in law is between powers and duties. At first sight, the difference is fairly clear – legislation which says that a local authority 'can' or 'may' do something is giving a power, whereas if it uses the terms 'shall' or 'must', then it is imposing a duty.

Local authorities may not do things that they are not legally empowered to do. That would be to act *ultra vires*, beyond their powers, and could be challenged in the courts. Even if they do have a power to decide or do something, local authorities still do not have a free rein. They must consider the duties that they have (including those in other legislation, such as the Equality Act 2010), and especially the requirements of the ECHR. They must also follow the regulations and guidance issued by the government, and the standard principles of administrative justice (i.e. legality, fairness, rationality and proportionality, discussed further below).

Statutory duties fall into two main categories, individual duties and general duties. Individual duties, also known as specific duties, bring enforceable rights to the person to whom the duty is owed. Therefore, if the person considers that the duty has not been carried out, they could take the council to court (for example, if they consider they have been denied a service to which they are entitled). General duties, also known as target duties, are worded in broad terms and do not bring individual entitlements. An example is s. 17 of the Children Act 1989:

> s. 17(1): It shall be the general duty of every local authority . . .
> (a) to safeguard and promote the welfare of children within their area who are in need; and
> (b) in so far as is consistent with that duty, to promote the upbringing of such children by their families,
> by providing a range and level of services appropriate to those children's needs.

There is no specific entitlement here to any services for any individual child. Local authorities are expected to work with other relevant agencies (other statutory services, voluntary organisations and private enterprises) to ensure that there is a suitable range of services to meet the variety of needs of children and families in their area. Under s. 10 of the Children Act 2004, local authorities have a responsibility to work with other agencies to improve the well-being of *all* children in their area, not only those who meet the criteria of being in need under s. 17 of the 1989 Act.

Even when the law appears to impose specific duties, it is often set about with qualifying phrases, such as 'as appears to them reasonable', or 'in so far as is practicable'. These are not an excuse not to try, and the decision that a course of action is not reasonable or practicable must be based on sound reasoning, properly authorised and clearly recorded; but legal duties are often not as absolute as they may seem at first.

A main reason why a local authority may not always consider it reasonable to meet a particular need, is the cost of the service(s) balanced against the overall level of demand and the availability of resources. From an ethical perspective, we can see it as an example of utilitarian reasoning, the need to restrict the benefits for one person in order to spread the resources among others, to get the greatest good for the greatest number.

The leading case is *R v Gloucestershire County Council ex parte Barry* [1997]. Mr Barry had been receiving community care services under s. 2(1) of the Chronically Sick and Disabled Persons Act 1970 (CSDPA). This imposes a specific duty on the local authority to arrange certain welfare services for a disabled person, if they are satisfied that it is necessary to make those arrangements in order to meet his needs. However, the courts have held that even though this is a specific duty, it does not mean that resources are not relevant.

In the Barry case, the authority decided it had to reduce its community care services because of financial constraints. It wrote to 1,500 service users to cut their services. Mr Barry and others applied for judicial review (this procedure is discussed below). Eventually the matter got as far as the House of Lords. The decision, by a majority of 3–2, was that local authorities can take account of resources when assessing someone's needs and in deciding whether or not to provide services, but must not change a care package without reassessing the person's situation. There is a three-stage process. The first step is to assess the need. Here, as subsequent guidance has clarified, there is a difference between the 'presenting need' and the 'eligible need'. The latter does take account of the authority's resources (DH, 2003; updated DH, 2010b). The second step is deciding how best to meet the eligible needs. Again, resources can be taken into account. The third step is to provide the services. The authority cannot change the services without a reassessment of the person's needs. (For helpful commentaries on this case, see Laird, 2010: 353–60; Clements and Thompson, 2011: 99–110.)

Principles of decision-making

When making decisions about how to exercise their powers and fulfil their duties, public bodies must act lawfully. The key aspects are legality, fairness, rationality and proportionality.

In terms of legality, public bodies must obey the law about what they do or do not do, and in the way they reach decisions. Even where they appear to have discretion, they must follow public law principles about decision-making. The aim of these is to ensure fairness and rationality. For example, the authority must take due account of relevant information, and not be swayed by irrelevant information; they must take reasonable steps to gather the information they need (e.g. commissioning reports from other agencies or appropriate experts; having review processes); and they must not fetter their own discretion by applying a policy very rigidly, as though it were a law. They must uphold people's 'legitimate expectations' (e.g. if they have made a promise, they must keep it). They have to show that they have acted fairly, for example by ensuring that the decision-makers do not have any vested interest in a particular outcome, and by ensuring that the individual(s) concerned know the case against them and have the opportunity to prepare and put forward their reply.

The notion of rationality, or reasonableness, is captured in the *Wednesbury* principles, named after a legal case called *Associated Provincial Picture Houses v Wednesbury Corporation* [1947]. The principles require that public authorities consider all relevant matters and exclude all irrelevant ones; but even if the authority has done this, if the decision it has reached is judged so unreasonable that no reasonable authority could ever have reached it, the court will still be able to overturn it. This is, however, a very high test to meet. The ECHR means that nowadays the authority must also consider the notion of proportionality, which is a different set of considerations, and more intense than reasonableness.

The test of proportionality applies when the matter involves an ECHR right, such as the right to private and family life (Article 8). It requires the authority (or court) to balance the general interests of society and the legitimate aims of the state, against the rights and interests of the individual. The questions that have to be asked are whether the decision or action is necessary and appropriate given the risks involved. Has the authority considered a less intrusive alternative? Do the ends really justify the means?

The courts offer an important route for individuals to challenge the way that public authorities exercise their powers and duties, through the procedure of *judicial review*. (Local authorities may also use it to challenge the decisions of central government.) This has become increasingly significant and used much more often in recent years, particularly since the ECHR was incorporated into UK law. The focus is not the decision itself, but whether the authority acted lawfully in reaching its decision. The courts will review this in terms of legality, fairness, rationality and proportionality (see Williams, 2010).

Judicial review is an important way of holding public authorities to account for their decision-making. However, there are three warning points to make. First, there are strict criteria about who can make a claim, and under what circumstances. The complaint has to be about the process of decision-making, not simply dissatisfaction with the decision (this could be dealt with by a complaint or an appeal, but not judicial review). The claimant has to show that they have sufficient interest in the matter, and they have to apply within three months of the decision. This is a very tight time limit given that claimants have to show they have tried other ways of dealing with the matter first, such as the authority's ordinary complaints procedures, a tribunal or the local government ombudsman. Nevertheless, the threat of judicial review has become a widespread strategy that lawyers use when arguing for their clients against local authorities.

The second point is that in judicial review, even if the court upholds the claimant's case, it ordinarily sends the matter back to the authority to consider the matter again, in the light of the court's judgment. This means that the authority could come to the same decision, but lawfully this time. Critics argue that this shows the limitations of judicial review. An authority might make procedural changes to safeguard itself from future challenge, but not improve its decision-making in any real sense (see Richardson, 2004, for a summary of UK research on the impact of judicial review). Sunkin *et al.* (2008) found that judgments can have a positive impact, but it is a complex terrain and many other factors come into play, notably organisational dynamics, high levels of demand and tight budgets. This leads to the third warning, which is that from the perspective of local authorities, the cost (in time and money) of responding to judicial reviews and repeated threats of review, can be highly disruptive to the overall level of service (Dickens, 2006).

Conclusion

This chapter has discussed the legal framework for social work in England in terms of the different sources of law (Parliament, the courts and the two European dimensions), the court structure, and the key distinctions between law and guidance, civil and criminal law, and powers and duties. It has also highlighted four crucial elements of lawful decision-making for public authorities.

For all the political debate, the tiers of courts and the principles of decision-making, laws and court judgments can sometimes feel unfair. This suggests that there are notions of fairness that lie beyond law. People have pre-existing understandings of justice, rights, duty, care and so on, and compare laws and court decisions to them. To what extent do our laws and court judgments match our moral values, and why might they sometimes be in conflict with them? This brings us to questions about morality and ethics, and we turn to those in more detail in Chapter 4.

Chapter 4

Questions for reflection

- Think about a family or individual service user you have worked with, and think about the four decision-making principles of legality, fairness, rationality and proportionality. How were you applying those principles in your work with them?

- Can you think of a law or a court decision which goes against your moral values? Try to think closely about why – what exactly are the grounds of your discomfort or disagreement?

Useful websites and further reading

The BAILII website (*British and Irish Legal Information Institute*) is a comprehensive database of court judgments from the UK and around the world: www.bailii.org.uk

European Court of Human Rights: www.echr.coe.int/echr/Homepage_EN

EU law is available via the *Europa* website: http://eur-lex.europa.eu/en/index.htm

UK Supreme Court (including a link to live coverage of the hearings – well worth watching): www.supremecourt.gov.uk

Community Care, the social work news and jobs website, gives useful updates on legislation and case law: www.communitycare.co.uk

As noted in Chapter 1, there is a good range of helpful textbooks about the law for social workers. As well as the three mentioned there, other useful books are:

- Barber, Brown and Martin (2012) *Mental Health Law in England and Wales*, 2nd edition.

- Braye and Preston-Shoot (2010) *Practising Social Work Law*, 3rd edition.

- Clements and Thompson (2011) *Community Care and the Law*, 5th edition.

- Davis (2009) *The Social Worker's Guide to Children and Families Law*.

- Hill (2010) *Working in Statutory Contexts*.

- Laird (2010) *Practical Social Work Law*.

- Long, Roche and Stringer (eds) (2010) *The Law and Social Work*, 2nd edition.

- Seymour and Seymour (2011) *Courtroom and Report Writing Skills for Social Workers*, 2nd edition.

- White, Broadbent and Brown (2009) *Law and the Social Work Practitioner*, 2nd edition.

- Williams (2008) *Child Law for Social Work*.

4 The ethical framework

This chapter introduces the ethical framework that shapes the discussions about social work and the law throughout the book. It describes four major western schools of thought about ethical codes and social values – Kantian, utilitarian, virtue and care. At first sight these may appear rather remote from contemporary social work practice, but not at all: the central question that they all address is how do we decide what to do, how do we evaluate the moral worth of a course of action? How important is our understanding of our duty (the Kantians), our assessment of the consequences (the utilitarians), our sense of what the good person would do (virtue ethics), or our feelings of care and the importance of relationships (care ethics)?

The overlaps and tensions between these four approaches make them central to political and social life in our modern, liberal democratic society. The chapter begins to draw out the implications for social work and its relationships with law. These will be developed further in the following chapters. The central message is to appreciate the strengths and limitations of all four approaches, and to use them in a creative, interactive way, to evaluate, challenge and refine one another (Houston, 2011, also takes this approach).

The chapter is a basic introduction to the ethical approaches, referring to selected key texts. All of them have their own history of debates and re-interpretations, and variants within them. The reading list at the end of the chapter should be useful to readers who wish to explore the ethical background in greater detail. The main features of the approaches are summarised in Table 4.1.

Table 4.1
Four ethical approaches

Ethical approach	Kantian (Deontology)	Utilitarian	Virtue	Care
Core concept	Duty	'Utility' – the greatest happiness principle	Character	Relationships
Understanding of individuals and society	Individuals are autonomous moral agents. Their moral responsibility is to 'do the right thing', regardless of the consequences.	Individuals are autonomous moral agents. Their moral responsibility is to do what has the best consequences for society as whole.	Individuals have a moral responsibility to live a virtuous life, doing the right thing for the right reasons. Virtues are learned and practised in the society to which people belong.	An individual's moral identity and responsibility is shaped by their personal relationships with others.
Understanding of reason and emotions	Rationality enables humans to determine their duty. They must do this, categorically. Reason, not emotions and feelings, is the mainspring of morality.	Reason is used to translate human emotions and desires, notably the desire for happiness, into mainsprings of morality.	Rationality is a key virtue, but cannot be isolated from practical virtues such as courage, empathy, generosity.	Rationality is less important than key interpersonal values of love, care, concern (but there is still a role for it).
Implications for social work policy and practice	The foundation of traditional social work values for working with individuals, such as respect, honesty and confidentiality.	The foundation of traditional social work values for working on behalf of society, such as fairness and social well-being.	The foundation of traditional social work values for working with individuals, such as integrity and kindness.	The foundation of traditional social work values for working with individuals in relationship-based practice.
Approach to the law	Laws and courts important to ensure freedom for individuals and equality.	Laws and courts important to ensure overall well-being of society.	Laws and courts important to create the conditions for people to become virtuous.	Laws and courts less relevant, and sometimes harmful to complex human relationships of trust, loyalty, love.

Kantian approaches: the search for categorical answers

Immanuel Kant lived from 1724 to 1804 in the city of Konigsberg, East Prussia (now Kaliningrad). He was a philosopher of the Enlightenment, 'the age of reason', when new ideas about science and the role of human beings in creating and ordering their own world were taking hold. These challenged old ways of thinking that the world and society were created and ordered by God, operating according to divine laws, and that moral behaviour was a matter of following God-given rules. For Kant, rules about proper conduct, duties, are not imposed by God, but created by humans, using their reason – but the thorough and consistent application of reason to any given situation will produce binding laws. Kant thought that the application of 'pure practical reason' – that is, logical thinking (pure reason) about moral matters (practical reason) – would come up with the same rules every time, giving universal laws. So humans do end up following moral rules, things they must do, categorically, but these are the products of their own rational thought, freely imposed upon themselves. Kant was also arguing against the utilitarians (see below), who shared the Enlightenment approach to human agency, but had a very different view about the relationship between reason and human desires or self-interest.

In *The Foundation* (or *Groundwork*) *of the Metaphysics of Morals* (1785), Kant starts by saying that the only thing that can be considered 'good' is a good will. Other personal qualities, for example courage, could easily be used for bad purposes; the only thing that ensures they are put to good ends is a good will. So what makes a good will?

Kant proposes that it is made through the thorough and consistent application of reason in accordance with a 'categorical imperative', an overall principle that *has* to be followed. It is categorical, it is our duty, and Kantian ethics are the leading example of a 'deontological', or duty-based approach. Kant gives different formulations of the categorical imperative, but the best-known two are:

- Act only on that maxim whereby thou canst at the same time will that it should become a universal law;

- So act as to treat humanity, whether in thine own person or in that of any other, in every case as an end, never as a means only.

(Kant, 1785: Section 2, paras 39 and 59)

The language may be old-fashioned but the central ideas are clear enough. The first version is that, in any situation, we should only act in such a way that we could wish that everyone else would behave that way in those circumstances. One of Kant's examples is giving a false promise in order to borrow money. Could we wish that it became a universal law, that whenever someone needs a loan, they can make a promise that they will repay it, but not intending to do so? Kant's answer is that we obviously cannot; but it is important to appreciate that for Kant this is not because of the consequences, but because of the logical inconsistency. We simply cannot have a situation where a promise is defined as an undertaking to do something, *and* we allow people to make promises without intending to do what they say. It would make the whole notion of promising meaningless.

For Kant the problem with a false promise is not (say) that the banks will run out of money if everyone acts this way. That might be a consequence, but Kant is not a consequentialist – for him, an action is right or wrong according to the motives for which it is done, not the results. If it is done according to the categorical imperative then it is morally worthy, and the results are irrelevant. Equally, even if an act has good results, it should not be considered moral if it was not done for the right reasons – if, for example (turning now to the second version of the categorical imperative), the act treats a person as a means not an end. One of Kant's examples is a shopkeeper who gives the correct change to a child, even though he could short-change him. It is the right thing to do, but if the shopkeeper's motivation is to get a good business reputation, then it does not have moral worth.

The example of the shopkeeper raises a problem for Kant's duty-based approach. Does something have moral worth *only* if it is done out of a sense of duty? Say the shopkeeper realises that he could short-change the child, but does not do so because it gives him pleasure to do the right thing, makes him feel good to know he is the sort of person who treats all his customers fairly. So he has not acted out of sense of duty, but because of personal satisfaction and pleasure. Has that invalidated any claim to moral value?

Kant recognises that human interests and desires do a play a part in motivating action, but his argument against the utilitarians is that these are not the basis of morality and moral action. For Kant, there are two worlds, the physical world of the senses and desires, and the world of reason and understanding. Human beings are part of both, but the physical world constrains people, and only in the world of reason is one free – and one has to be free to act truly morally. This can seem a hard message. Many helpful people might say they enjoy helping others. A feeling of satisfaction from helping people is likely to be a motivating factor for most social workers in choosing their career. Kant's emphasis on rationality and self-imposed duty can sometimes seem to undervalue an important aspect of human character.

Kant's approach to the law is that it should allow the maximum amount of freedom for all people consistent with these principles. This is his 'universal law of justice'. Putting it simply, the idea is that we should treat other people the way that we would (logically) wish to be treated ourselves, as ends not only means, and in accordance with rules that apply to all. The law should reflect and uphold this approach. It should allow people to use their own reason and reach their own decisions, and only allow intervention when necessary to protect the person and others.

Utilitarianian approaches: weighing the consequences

In modern everyday language, the term 'utilitarian' has come to mean something functional and rather dull – to describe a building as utilitarian, for example, is to be rather disparaging about it, to portray it as a cheerless design. However, utilitarianism has a long history as an approach to ethics based on understandings of human happiness and well-being, not dull functionality. The ideas were popularised by Jeremy Bentham in his *Introduction to the Principles of Morals and Legislation* (1780). Kant was arguing against Bentham's views. Later, John Stuart Mill would take up the debate and refine Bentham's ideas in his work, *Utilitarianism* (1861). The utilitarians share Kant's belief in the importance of reason, but they do not see it as a separate sphere to humans' own interests and desires. On the contrary, rationality must take account of these wishes and *use* them in the way that moral standards and laws are set and upheld.

Utilitarianism is a consequentialist approach, holding that the moral worth of an action depends on its outcomes. The well-known catchphrase is whether it produces 'the greatest happiness for the greatest number', although there are other versions such as the 'greatest good' for the greatest number, or the 'greatest welfare'. Whatever the formulation, similar issues arise, such as the difficulties of defining and measuring happiness, the good or welfare, and whether it is acceptable to overrule the interests of an individual in order to secure the greatest benefits.

In *Utilitarianism*, Mill explains the approach as follows:

> Utility, or the Greatest-Happiness Principle, holds that actions are right in proportion as they tend to promote happiness, wrong as they tend to produce the reverse of happiness. By happiness is intended pleasure, and the absence of pain; by unhappiness, pain, and the privation of pleasure.
>
> (Mill, 1861: Chap. 2, para. 2)

The point for utilitarians is that most people *do* look for their own happiness – gaining pleasure and avoiding pain is a guiding principle for most people, most of the time (Mill does not just mean physical pleasures). Given that this is a fact of human nature, the goal of education and legislation should be to promote behaviour that enables people to achieve happiness for themselves *and* the happiness of the whole.

As Mill (1861: Chap. 2, para. 9) puts it, 'the standard is not the agent's own greatest happiness, but the greatest amount of happiness altogether'. On this basis, then, it is legitimate to punish someone for a crime, say by sending them to prison, even though that may inflict pain and reduce pleasure for them, because it increases the happiness of the majority by preventing crime and maintaining social order. (Ideas about crime and punishment are discussed more fully in Chapter 10.) There are three major areas of difficulty for utilitarianism.

Motives and consequences

For utilitarians, the test of morality is the consequences of an action – does it increase the general happiness or not? Stealing something might increase the individual wrong-doer's happiness, but it is unlikely to increase the overall happiness of society, so therefore it is, usually, wrong (although in some circumstances it may be acceptable – see further below). Mill argues that the motive an individual has for doing something does not affect the morality of the *action* (that depends on the consequences) although it does reveal a great deal about the moral worthiness of the individual. For Kant, of course, moral worth lies in the motive, not the consequences. So, both approaches seek to distinguish between motives and consequences, but they put the weight on different sides. It is certainly an important distinction, but whether one can evaluate the moral worth of an action without reference to both seems unlikely; but then, of course, the challenge is to find a suitable balance between the two. (The relationship between motives and consequences is discussed again in Chapter 9, when considering the question of social workers' responsibility for poor outcomes in their cases.)

Individuals and society

What if the general happiness could be increased by committing a crime, or even by imprisoning an innocent person? Perhaps someone who is a bit different, or an eccentric, rather than someone who is guilty; or someone who is suspected of an offence, or even merely thought likely to commit an offence, rather than someone who actually has? Utilitarianism seems to justify the trading-off of an individual's interests against the greater interests of society as a whole. Mill puts it this way:

> to save a life it may not only be allowable, but a duty, to steal, or take by force, the necessary food or medicine, or to kidnap, or compel to officiate, the only qualified medical practitioner.
>
> (Mill, 1861: Chap. 5, para. 37)

For utilitarians, the general position, the rule, is that an innocent person should not go to prison, and that people should not steal food or medicine. Generally it is best to obey such rules, because society and the law would be undermined if innocent people were detained, and if stealing were allowed just because people needed the items. People's trust in their government and the law would fall and the end result would be worse for all, a mistrustful and unhappy society. Also, in reality we do not have the time or the knowledge to weigh up all the advantages and disadvantages of breaking the normal rule, so it is generally best to stick to the tried and tested standards; but still, utilitarianism allows the possibility that in certain circumstances, albeit extreme, the normal rules can be overruled. The danger is that an individual's rights could be badly infringed – perhaps, the person could be tortured.

At this point it is useful to refer to another of Mill's works, *On Liberty* (1859). Here, he argues that whilst he regards utility as the 'the ultimate appeal on all ethical questions', it must be 'utility in the largest sense'. Generally, this is best served by the highest degree of individual freedom, and the only reason to compel someone to act against their own will should be to prevent harm to others. The individual's

own good is not a sufficient warrant. So Mill sets high value on individual freedom, alongside his utilitarianism (indeed, as part of his utilitarianism); but in some circumstances individual freedoms may be restricted. Different dimensions of freedom are discussed further in Chapter 5.

Utilitarianism raises profound practical challenges for social work. Social workers will often come across dilemmas when the needs and rights of one person have to balance against the needs and rights of others. These could be situations where one person's behaviour creates risks for others, or when hard decisions have to be made about how best to use limited resources. Social workers may also intervene when a person's behaviour places their own welfare at risk. These situations do not justify disregarding the person's rights, but may justify overruling them, provided proper safeguards and processes are followed.

What is happiness?

A further difficulty for utilitarianism is about the nature of happiness, and whether happiness really is the ultimate value. Surely some things are more important – honesty, courage, kindness, for example – and surely, not all sorts of pleasure are equally worthy? As noted earlier, similar questions arise even if we talk about the greatest good, or welfare – what counts, and who judges? For Bentham, all pleasures counted the same if they gave the same quantity of happiness – he claimed that 'pushpin is as good as poetry' (pushpin was a child's game). That seems to miss a great deal of what it is to be human, taking on the challenges and pains of working for high standards rather than settling for the easiest option.

Mill disagrees with Bentham, and argues that it is better to be Socrates dissatisfied than a fool satisfied; and if the fool disagrees, that's because he's a fool and only knows his own side of the story. But to claim that pleasures can be graded, and some are higher than others, cuts at the heart of utilitarianism. It suggests that there is an external standard against which happiness has to be judged – it is not enough just to be satisfied, you have to be satisfied about the right things. But if that is the case, then happiness is no longer the sole criterion for morality. It seems that after all we do have to look towards other standards, such as categorical approaches or virtue-based accounts.

Virtue-based approaches: the importance of character

Rather than look for moral rules to guide behaviour, virtue-based accounts look at the qualities of character that a 'virtuous' person has, and take these as a guide to moral behaviour. The most famous example is Aristotle's *Nicomachean Ethics* (named after his son, Nicomachus), written in 350 BCE. Virtue-based ethics have become popular approaches recently in social work and social care, explored well in Banks and Gallagher (2009) (and see Rhodes, 1986; McBeath and Webb, 2002; Houston, 2003; Clark, 2006a; Banks, 2010).

For Aristotle, the chief good in life, the ultimate goal or 'end' of all human endeavour, is *eudaimonia*, which is often translated as 'well-being', or 'flourishing'. It is sometimes translated as 'happiness', which brings out the similarities and differences to utilitarianism. How can people achieve well-being, or true happiness? The answer is that it comes through virtuous living (not from weighing up pleasures and pains, or just following duty). This is the result of education and training. It is not enough just to know what is right, to have theoretical knowledge of the good life, virtuous living has to become a matter of habit. One has to do the right thing out of inclination (not, as Kant holds, against inclination). People acquire the virtues by *doing* them. At first we may only act the right way because we are told to, or through fear, or even by luck; but over time, through repetition, our understanding of the virtues and ability to act accordingly becomes part of our character – we become virtuous people. Virtues are states of character, dispositions, but they are acquired through education and action, not inherited, and they have to be put into practice. By doing them we become more likely to do them (a virtuous circle). The law has a part to play in this too, because the purpose of legislation is to help citizens form good habits.

Aristotle distinguishes between intellectual and moral virtues, but ultimately all are inter-related. His list of moral virtues includes courage, moderation, liberality and sincerity. The intellectual virtues include contemplation (the ability to reflect on the ultimate, unchanging truths of life), and knowledge (needed to cope with the changing aspects of life). For Aristotle, contemplation is the highest virtue because it brings the greatest happiness, or well-being. However, it is crucial to Aristotle's approach that the intellectual and moral virtues are intertwined. The intellectual virtues tell us what to do, give us the principles of action; the moral ones enable us to do it.

Aristotle defines the moral virtues with his 'doctrine of the mean'. That is to say, courage can be distinguished from cowardice and also from rashness – it is the mean, in the middle, between two extremes. Too much bravery, in certain circumstances, can be as harmful as too little in another situation. Similarly, moderation lies between self-indulgence and self-denial, liberality between meanness and wastefulness. But exactly what counts as courageous, moderate or liberal depends on the particular circumstances, so the virtues are context-bound. That is why we cannot have absolute rules about behaviour, but have to use reason, the intellectual virtues, and draw on experience, the habits of moral virtue.

There is a second sense in which Aristotle's virtues are context-bound. They are not just dependent on the specifics of a situation, they are closely linked with the community in which they are formed, practised and valued. They do not include the traditional 'Christian virtues' of kindness and humility, for example: Aristotle's virtues are the virtues of an Athenian aristocrat in the fourth century BCE, and inseparable from the life of the Athenian city-state (MacIntyre, 1985). Of course, this creates some problems for virtue ethics, because it raises the thorny issue of how to decide what counts as a virtue. Different communities may have different views, and different groups within a community may have different views too. Houston (2003) debates this problem, and argues that virtue has to be defined through dialogue between all the parties involved. Drawing on Habermas' theory of discourse ethics, he paints a demanding but inspiring picture of how this dialogue should operate. It must be 'an unremitting quest to empathize with perspectives that are different to my own'; and it should proceed 'on the basis of inclusivity, open communication, empathy, and impartiality' (Houston, 2003: 823).

As for the relationship between ethics and the law, Aristotle sees the role of the state, through legislation, to create the conditions for people to act virtuously. For some people, this will become habitual, part of their character; for others (the majority) punishments and penalties will be needed to encourage them. Aristotle argues that the highest aim for an individual should be to become capable of legislating, to play their part in political debate and decision-making. The *Nicomachean Ethics* ends with a call to study political constitutions, laws and customs, because it is only through understanding what makes a successful community that one can truly understand human nature and how to help individuals achieve well-being.

Even after almost two and a half thousand years, Aristotle's ethics carries challenging messages for us today. It has particular implications for social work, where the notion of the worker's moral character is crucial. Social workers are required (amongst other things) to be honest and trustworthy; reliable and dependable; not to form inappropriate personal relationships with service users; and not to behave in a way 'in work or outside work, which would call into question your suitability to work in social care services' (GSCC, 2002a).

Virtue ethics show us that it is not enough merely to know what is good, we have understand it and *do* it, all the time; and despite the widespread, modern understanding of virtues as individual character traits, Aristotle's approach teaches us that they are things that can be learned, and are not just a private matter, but inextricably linked to public life and social responsibilities.

Care ethics: the importance of relationships

Care ethics is our fourth model of ethical thinking and action, although it is important to recognise that there are distinct but related approaches within this broad heading (Meagher and Parton, 2004; Held, 2006; Gray, 2010; Featherstone, 2010). Rather than relying on reason, happiness or virtue to tell us what to do, care ethics emphasises the centrality of caring human relationships as the grounding for moral behaviour.

Two writers played the leading roles in the origins of care ethics, Carol Gilligan (1982) and Nel Noddings (2003, 1st edition 1984). Taking Noddings' work to illustrate the themes, the focus is on private, family relationships, particularly the mother–child relationship, and the close emotional bonds of love and care. For Noddings, it is a distinctively feminine approach. That is not to say that men cannot show love and care too (or that all women necessarily do), but that the key features of care ethics are more characteristically and essentially feminine (Noddings, 2003: 8). Noddings identifies the key features as receptivity, relatedness and responsiveness to the other person. She rejects the 'male' approach of rationality, rigid rules and universal principles, and emphasises the need to respond sensitively and flexibly to each person's unique needs and circumstances.

Noddings values intuition, feelings and the innate imperative to care. So, for example, unlike Kant who holds that it is never right to tell a lie, Noddings argues that it may be acceptable to tell lies out of care for the person concerned. The example she gives is of a mother who decides to take her child out of school for a day to do something worthwhile together. Afterwards, the mother writes a letter to the school to say that her child was ill, because otherwise the child would be given detention (Noddings, 2003: 56–7). It may seem a simple example, but it raises many hard questions. What message is the mother giving to her child? And what if things were slightly different, and the child had refused to go to school – should the mother tell a lie then? How many lies, and what sort of lies, is a mother allowed to tell for her child? What if she thinks her child has committed a serious offence? These are uncomfortable questions, but Noddings' point is that ethical decisions are not made by ascertaining universal rules, but by following an ideal of caring in specific situations. However, Noddings asserts that thinking has its place too. It is not simply a matter of following the emotions, and she insists on a 'clear-eyed inspection of our feelings, longings, fears, hopes, dreams' (2003: 57).

The three key elements of Noddings' approach – femininity, close family relationships as the model for moral behaviour, and the contrast with principle-based approaches – have, inevitably, been highly controversial, and alternative approaches to care ethics have been developed (notably Tronto, 1993; Sevenhuijsen, 2000; Williams, 2001). Instead of a *feminine* ethics of care, alternative approaches speak of a *feminist* ethics of care. The distinction is that instead of focusing on purported 'essential' differences between men and women, a feminist approach is a critique of the ways of thinking that elevate certain values and ways of behaving over others, and in the process demean those that are seen as more feminine. So, for example, values that are often seen as masculine, such as rationality, independence and justice are prized above others that are often characterised as feminine (emotion, interdependency, care). Both sexes get stereotyped and bound into particular ways of behaving, but the cost is much greater to women.

Further, instead of a narrowly interpersonal model of caring relationships, alternative approaches highlight the public, political and policy aspects of care. For Williams (2001), a *political* ethics of care is a counter to the 'ethic of paid work' that was so important in the welfare policies of the New Labour government of 1997–2010 (and continues to be central to current government policy). Sevenhuijsen (2000) is also highly critical of the dominance of an oppressive work ethic, arguing that politics and policy must recognise the importance of caring in society and the values that come with it – core values of attentiveness, responsibility, competence, responsiveness and integrity (drawing on Tronto, 1993). And rather than seeing a care ethic and a justice ethic as separate and incompatible, feminist care ethics sees them as balancing and reframing one another. Each is essential. There is a dark side to care, that it can be exceptionally demanding of the carer, and also very controlling of the person cared-for. Both dangers need a notion of justice to counter-balance them, a framework of rights and empowerment (Meagher and Parton, 2004; Lloyd, 2006; Gray, 2010). Equally, formal justice, such as legal processes, can be insensitive to the needs of individuals. An ethics of care can ameliorate the law's narrow views, its tendency to reduce complex matters to simple questions of admissible or not admissible, guilty or not guilty.

Care is at the heart of social work, even though it may often be in tension with other imperatives, such as working for change and the enforcement of social control. Social workers may work as 'care managers', assessing needs and arranging individual budgets or commissioning services. Social workers may work with children in care (Holland, 2010), or with people who are carers. The term 'care' is

 ubiquitous, and although the image of interpersonal caring relationships accounts for some of the ways it is used in social work, it certainly does not capture them all. The public policy aspects and the law come into play too, as we saw in the discussion about the 'duty of care' in Chapter 2.

Chapter 2

Conclusion

This chapter has summarised four major ethical approaches that give a framework for debating and analysing the interactions of law, ethics and social work. It has shown how all four approaches are wrestling with the questions of how the individual relates to society, and how to balance freedom and control. For Kant, the individual comes first; for Mill, society (but a society that prizes individual freedom); for Aristotle, the individual in social context; and for care ethics, the individual in relationships. There are differences and overlaps between the various schools, and dynamic interaction between them is a key to creative and rigorous ethical thinking. The next chapter offers further perspectives on the relationships between the individual and society, freedom and control.

A new key pairing has emerged through the chapter, reason and emotion. The three older schools of thought all emphasise rationality above intuition. For Kantians, instincts and feelings are considered unreliable and misleading. We have to put our intellect first, using it to work out what our duty is, and applying it. For utilitarians, feelings of pleasure or pain are a starting point for ethical behaviour, but we must not be misled by our own emotions. We always have to weigh up how our actions will affect the overall happiness. For virtue approaches, our instincts must be trained, through education and socialisation, to help us behave in the ways of a person of good character. Care ethics has a different approach. Here, our feelings and emotions are the foundation of ethical conduct, but even so we need to use our reason to assess those feelings. The balance of reason and emotion is another crucial dimension for thinking about the interaction of social work, law and ethics.

Questions for reflection

- What matters more for the moral worth of an action – the motives or the consequences? Explain your thinking.

- Consider again the differences between a feminine and a feminist ethic of care. Which do you think is the more convincing, and what are your reasons?

Useful websites and further reading

Sandel (2009) *Justice: What's the Right Thing to Do?* Michael Sandel's Harvard University lecture course, *Justice*, is available online, at www.justiceharvard.org. You can download and watch his lectures on (amongst others) Kant, utilitarianism and Aristotle. They are clear and very enjoyable.

The classic texts referred to in this chapter, by Kant, Mill and Aristotle, are all available online.

Principles and frameworks

There is a good range of textbooks on ethics and values for social work. Leading introductions to the subject are:

- Banks (2004) *Ethics, Accountability and the Social Professions.*

- Banks (2012) *Ethics and Values in Social Work*, 4th edition.

- Banks and Gallagher (2009) *Ethics in Professional Life.*

- Barnard, Horner and Wild (eds) (2008) *The Value Base of Social Work and Social Care.*

- Beckett and Maynard (2005) *Values and Ethics in Social Work: An Introduction.*

- Gray and Webb (eds) (2010) *Ethics and Value Perspectives in Social Work.*

- Hugman (2005) *New Approaches in Ethics for the Caring Professions.*

- Parrott (2006) *Values and Ethics in Social Work Practice.*

5 Freedom and society

One of the powerful themes in Chapter 4 is that ethics are not just matters of individual decisions and behaviour, but are interwoven with social values and social living. Our codes of behaviour are learned

Chapters 4 & 1

from others and with others, put into practice in social contexts, and have consequences for other individuals and for society in general. This goes back to one of the key pairings discussed in Chapter 1, the relationship between the individual and society. This chapter adds more angles to that topic, linking it with ideas about freedom and the role of the law.

'Freedom' is one of the core values in western societies – freedom for individuals to live their lives as they see fit, except for certain restrictions to safeguard the freedoms of others and to protect vulnerable people from the most harmful consequences of their own decisions. But there are different views about how much freedom is appropriate, and what sort of freedom. The first part of the chapter describes four different approaches to freedom, where ethics interweaves with politics and law, summarised in Table 5.1. There is freedom from undue state control (libertarianism), from poverty and social oppression (radicalism), freedom of diversity and to enjoy one's culture (relativism), and freedom to become oneself, to be truly authentic (existentialism).

The second part considers two questions about the role of law in society. The first is whether the law is of primary or secondary importance in creating and preserving an orderly society, and the second whether it serves the interests of society as a whole, or only those of the better-off. Views that see a generally benign role for law are known as consensus approaches. Those that see the law as imposing greater control on poorer people, keeping them down and 'in their place', are known as conflict approaches.

Freedom

Libertarianism

Libertarianism is a political philosophy that places greatest value on the maximum amount of individual freedom, and the minimum amount of state control. It mistrusts the state, arguing that it restricts individual initiative, undermines individual responsibility, is cumbersome, expensive and ineffective. Libertarians go a step beyond the liberalism of John Stuart Mill's essay *On Liberty* (1859), but it is a broad school and the term 'libertarian' includes very different approaches to social and economic freedoms.

For Mill, utility is the ultimate appeal on all ethical questions (as discussed in Chapter 4), but utility in the broadest sense, which is the overall interests of all citizens. In *On Liberty* Mill argues that this means the least amount of external control over an individual necessary to ensure the general welfare of others. Mill writes that 'the only purpose for which power can be rightfully exercised over any member of a civilised community, against his will, is to prevent harm to others. His own good, either physical or moral, is not a sufficient warrant ... Over himself, over his own body and mind, the individual is sovereign' (Mill, 1859: Chap. 1, para. 9).

Chapter 4

Having said that, Mill does allow for government intervention (and social pressure) to force individuals to act in certain ways, for the benefit of all. This includes punishing those who have harmed others (either through the courts or social disapproval), but also requires positive acts such as paying taxes, giving evidence in court, doing military service if required, and helping others whenever possible. So Mill is not an out-and-out libertarian, but is better regarded as a liberal. In broad terms, libertarians and liberals agree on the importance of individual freedom, but libertarians argue that this means a much reduced role for the state, whereas liberals see more positive potential for the state to promote and protect individual freedoms.

There are important differences between right and left wing versions of libertarianism. The right wing versions advocate high amounts of economic freedom (for example, low taxes, limited planning regulations, few if any constraints on international trade) but tend to be socially conservative. That is to say, they are not so keen on people being free to have 'alternative' lifestyles – not to have a job, to have children outside a stable relationship, to use recreational drugs. Modern forms of this right wing, economic version are often called 'neo-liberal', but this should not be confused with traditional social liberalism. Despite its rhetoric about liberty, it is a much less tolerant approach. The left wing versions of libertarianism are more likely to defend social freedoms and are less enthusiastic about economic deregulation, seeing this as socially dangerous and divisive.

Table 5.1
Four approaches to freedom

Approach	Libertarian	Radical	Relativist	Existentialist
Core concept of freedom	Freedom from overbearing state control.	Freedom from inequality and oppression.	Freedom for people to enjoy their own culture, to celebrate diversity.	Freedom to choose and to change, to be truly 'authentic'.
Understanding of individuals and society	Individuals are autonomous moral agents. Their moral responsibility is to provide for themselves and their families.	An individual's moral identity and responsibility is shaped by their social class and economic background. Societal responses are required to social problems, rather than blame and individualised action.	An individual's moral identity and responsibility is shaped by their cultural background. Different communities may have different values, but all should be respected.	Individuals are autonomous moral agents. Their moral responsibility is to fulfil themselves, decide what to do each time according to their own understanding and wishes, not to follow rules.
Understanding of reason and emotions	Rationality based on core notions of individual freedom and market-place principles. No room for sentimentality.	Rationality based on an understanding of the ways that economic and social systems (local and global) create and sustain inequality.	Reason is important to promote tolerance and mutual understanding. Recognises people's emotional ties to their own culture, and the psychological impact of being discriminated against.	Reason is important but so too are feelings. The goal is to be authentic, recognising one's freedom and living accordingly.
Implications for social work policy and practice	Underpins a reduced role for the state and welfare services – the state's role is to uphold people's independence and not intervene except when essential.	Underpins a greater role for state and welfare services – to maximise opportunities for people, especially those who are disadvantaged or discriminated against.	Underpins a commitment to culturally competent practice, and to anti-oppressive polices and practice.	Underpins a counselling and empowering role for social work, respecting people's individuality and enabling them to make their own decisions.
Approach to the law	Laws and courts should preserve individual freedoms. Also mistrustful of them for interfering too much and restricting individual liberties.	Laws and courts should ensure high-quality services and equality. At the same time, mistrustful of them for upholding the status quo.	Laws and courts should promote diversity and protect minority groups. Mistrustful of them for often failing to do this, being oppressive.	Laws and courts largely irrelevant, or seen as oppressive of individual freedom.

Radicalism

The word 'radical' comes from the Latin word for root, and so means to get to the roots, the bottom of something. In political discourse, it means a revolutionary, rather than a more steady, reformist approach – a radical approach offers a fundamental analysis of society and wants to see dramatic change. In that sense, both versions of libertarianism described above could be called radical; but in social work, the term radical is usually applied to left-wing, socialist approaches, and that is the sense in which it is used here (Bailey and Brake, 1975; Ferguson and Woodward, 2009; Lavalette, 2011; and see Weinberg, 2010).

Freedom from inequality and oppression is at the heart of radical, socialist philosophies. It is a very different view of freedom to the personal freedom of libertarianism, with its minimal role for the state. Karl Marx (1818–83) is historically the most prominent writer from this perspective, but people have always been aware of inequalities of wealth and opportunity, and there is a long history of protest and sometimes uprising about it (often put down very bloodily). The call for equality featured in the great revolutions of the eighteenth century. 'Liberty, Equality, Fraternity' was the slogan for the French Revolution, and the American Declaration of Independence asserts that 'all men are created equal' (we should insert 'and women'). Marx brought a new angle by grounding his analysis of inequality in the working of the capitalist economic system. For Marx, the fundamental distinction is between those who own the 'means of production' (e.g. businesses, factories, banks) and those who work for them. His ideas have been much revised, adapted, developed and argued over ever since.

Marxist perspectives on ethics, law and social work are important for the current book in two respects. First, they hold that all three are tools that the ruling class, the wealthy owners, use to subdue and control the working class. 'Morality' is the norms and values that they impose on poorer people, through education, training and employment, through the messages about 'responsible behaviour' conveyed in the popular media, and through the activities of welfare agencies such as housing departments, income support and social work. In these ways, beliefs about proper moral conduct become socially pervasive, controlling most people's thinking and behaviour, and isolating the non-conformists. They do not guarantee that everyone complies all the time (not even individual members of the ruling class, whose interests, as whole, the moral code serves) but the powerful messages preserve the social *status quo*, the way things are, and help to safeguard the position of the most powerful.

Marxists see the law and the courts operating in the same way. It is a conflict view, discussed further in the second part of this chapter, that the law serves the interests of the wealthy and the well connected. Occasionally the law may appear to uphold the rights of the 'little person' against the might of the state or a powerful corporation, but these tend to be small and isolated victories. Overall, law preserves the existing balance of power. And likewise social work: underneath the help that individual social workers may genuinely provide to individual service users, from a societal point of view the whole enterprise is more controlling than liberating.

But the second implication is this: despite the controlling aspects of morality, the law and state welfare, these can nevertheless be agents for social change and social justice. They are ambiguous, with the potential to liberate as well as to control. Law can protect the poor as well as the rich, and high-quality services can promote their welfare and empower them. Small changes can lead to bigger changes: and even small victories are worthwhile in themselves. An active state, and active individuals committed to social justice, can bring about a more equal society.

Cultural relativism

Chapters
2 & 11

Another face of freedom is the freedom to enjoy one's own culture, social traditions and choice of lifestyle. A commitment to anti-oppressive values and practice is a core requirement for professional social work, as noted in the discussion about equality in Chapter 2, and discussed further in Chapter 11. This means more than just being tolerant of differences between people such as culture, race, gender, sexuality, disability and age, but taking positive measures to challenge discrimination and disadvantages that arise from those differences.

From a relativist perspective, majority groups in society should not seek to impose their own values on people from other communities and other traditions, but should respect those differences. Legislation should be passed to protect minority groups, policies should be implemented to give them more equal opportunities, and welfare workers should be trained to recognise their strengths and respond to their needs in more culturally competent ways. In these respects, cultural relativism is a prime example of a liberal approach, seeing an important role for the state to ensure the well-being of all its citizens.

Whilst relativists welcome legislation and policies that defend and promote the rights of minority groups, they are also mistrustful of the ways that states, law and dominant ethical approaches can oppress minority or unconventional cultures, treating them as wrong, old-fashioned or themselves oppressive. A further dilemma for relativists is that there can be tensions between the imperative of valuing difference and the drive to tackle all forms of discrimination. Different cultural traditions about women's roles in society, sexuality and child discipline are prime examples. A liberal state will have laws to protect women, gay and lesbian people, and children – but sometimes those laws might be in tension with the principle of preserving cultural freedoms (see Healy, 2007).

Relativists are also ambivalent about the impact of international organisations and the international human rights discourse, exemplified in United Nations treaties such as the Convention on the Rights of the Child, or the Convention on the Rights of Persons with Disabilities. They welcome these in so far as they promote greater tolerance and support for minority cultures, but they are suspicious of the way that western understandings of families and society, of parenting, childhood and disability are being imposed on the rest of the world, devaluing different traditions and strengths. It is not that relativists condone ill-treatment of children or disabled people, but that they think the western nations ought to be more circumspect – it is not as though everything is rosy in their own garden.

The difficulty of extreme relativism is that it can be very conservative, against change, and can leave members of oppressed groups within a culture in very vulnerable positions. The relativists' answer is

Chapter 11

that rather than lecturing other nations and trying to impose their values, westerners ought to engage in cross-cultural dialogue, and support (but not interfere with) internal movements for change (An-Na'im, 1994, discussed in Chapter 11). They should aim to inspire change by being models of openness to debate and more equal ways of living, but not imposing solutions. Imposed solutions are, in any event, less likely to endure than changes that may take longer to achieve but come from within.

Similar principles apply within a country, to respect cultural differences and to resist imposing the values of the majority; but the challenges are more pressing when the same national legislation applies to all. There are hard decisions to be made about when it is reasonable to enforce certain requirements, when it is necessary to do so, the best tactics for achieving change and the limits of tolerance (Craig *et al.*, 2008).

Existentialism

Existentialist approaches place the highest value on individual freedom to choose. The most famous existentialist philosopher is Jean-Paul Sartre (1905–80). The implications of existentialism for social work have been developed helpfully by Neil Thompson (1992, 2000, 2008).

Existentialists recognise that there are great pressures from society and circumstances that can make people feel that they do not have real choices, that they are not truly free – social customs, rules, orders from people with more power than them, poverty, illness – but existentialists insist that individuals cannot hide behind these and deny their own responsibility for their decisions and their lives. To do so is 'bad faith'. People must accept their freedom and their responsibility. Their lives are not determined by external forces, their individual characteristics or even by 'human nature', if this is understood as something fixed and unchanging. Instead, people are always changing, becoming something new, and this openness to 'becoming' is what Sartre calls 'authenticity'.

Existentialism echoes Kantianism in its emphasis on individual responsibility and decision-making, but rejects the Kantian ideas of categorical rules that everyone should follow. On the contrary, each individual must decide for themselves in their own situation, and to say one was 'just following rules' is the highest form of bad faith. Nevertheless, one's decisions and actions do affect other people, and so one cannot ignore the social context and implications. For Sartre, individual freedom and responsibility must be the starting point for political freedom. The truly authentic person will question dominant values, will challenge the way that society is ordered. Sartre's existentialism leads to political action and social change.

Existentialism can seem a rather frightening approach, leaving each person on their own, having to decide for themselves, without the comfort of rules or the excuses of circumstances. On the other hand, this can be seen as truly liberating, breaking free from external constraints and false consciousness, and bringing the possibility of social as well as individual freedom.

There are echoes of existentialism in the way that modern social policy emphasises the centrality of service users' choices and self-determination. The role of public sector workers, including social workers, is often portrayed nowadays as an enabling and empowering one, helping service users to make their own decisions and achieve their own goals. In some respects this fits with an existentialist vision of society, and offers an exciting future for social work. Against this, many of the tasks that social workers undertake seem much more restricted than that, focused on managing risk, assessing need and commissioning services, more about control than freedom – but even so, the radical potential is there.

Law and society

The discussion about different aspects of freedom has raised further questions about the role of law in society – who it is for and what it is for, and how it links with ethics and social values.

In terms of law's social role, the notion of the 'rule of law' is central in western societies (see Box 5.1). The core ideas are that the laws of the land apply to everyone, not just citizens on the receiving end, but also to those who make and enforce them – to politicians, police officers, civil servants, judges, social workers and so on. The requirements of due process and transparency apply to all decisions, whether about individual cases or more general policy matters (see the principles of decision-making in Chapter 3).

Box 5.1: The rule of law

The United Nations defines the rule of law as:

> a principle of governance in which all persons, institutions and entities, public and private, including the State itself, are accountable to laws that are publicly promulgated, equally enforced and independently adjudicated, and which are consistent with international human rights norms and standards. It requires, as well, measures to ensure adherence to the principles of supremacy of law, equality before the law, accountability to the law, fairness in the application of the law, separation of powers, participation in decision-making, legal certainty, avoidance of arbitrariness and procedural and legal transparency.
>
> (UN, 2004: para. 6, available on the United Nations'
> 'rule of law' website: www.unrol.org)

The concept of the rule of law makes great claims for law's role in society (that law should rule, as opposed to tradition, religion, force, wealth, family connections and so on), but raises two sets of questions: first, is law really that important?

According to the rule of law approach, law is of primary importance for protecting people from arbitrary authority and unfairness, and for maintaining good social order. But as noted in the conclusion to Chapter 3, legislation and court judgments can sometimes feel unfair, showing that notions of fairness lie deeper than the law, however transparent and even-handed law making and law

enforcement may be. This suggests that law has only a secondary role in setting social standards. It might be necessary to uphold them, but does not form them. The 'heavy lifting' (Tonry, 2011: 384) is done elsewhere, by families, friends, communities, schools, religious groups and so on.

Law sceptics would argue that the limited usefulness of the law in deterring crime is an indication of its secondary role. Legal sanctions may deter some, but for most people law is not really that relevant to how they behave. For example, most people would not dream of stealing or committing assaults, whether or not these were against the law, or however severe the sentence was. Their values come first. Equally, others do commit such crimes, even though there are laws against them. This shows that law has a limited role in shaping individual character and conduct, and the values that are learned from families and communities come first. Unfortunately, these values may not always be the most robust or the most enlightened. It would be unwise to rely on them always to serve the interests of

vulnerable people and minority groups. Equally, it is unwise to rely on the law always to do that. Both sides are necessary, as Kant, Mill, Aristotle and the more politicised versions of care ethics all recognise (see Chapter 4). Which is on top is ambiguous and uncertain, and takes us back to the uneasy marriage analogy discussed in Chapter 1. Both have crucial parts to play in enforcing society's standards and challenging them when they are unfair.

Consensus and conflict

The second set of questions concern whether the rule of law really holds good – does the law really apply equally to all? There are two broad schools of thought about these questions, consensus and conflict. This is another important pairing for making sense of the social functions of law, and the relationship between law and ethics (see Hudson, 2003; Wacks, 2009; Travers, 2010; Tonry, 2011).

Consensus approaches hold that law helps society to run smoothly, reflecting and upholding social values. This is not to say that everything is agreed, or to deny that crimes occur and disputes arise, of course not: but it does hold that law helps to maintain social order and iron out difficult social problems and disputes. Law sets limits on what people can do and enforces control when necessary, in the interests of overall social well-being. It also gives individuals the powers to resist state intervention. It gives a secure framework for citizens to live their lives, based on individual rights and transparency about state powers. The underlying idea is that people accept certain limits on their

individual freedoms, in order to benefit from a stable and orderly society. Some freedoms need to be restricted in the interests of society as a whole (as the well-known saying puts it, 'freedom for the wolves is death to the lambs'). This 'social contract' approach has long historical roots, going back to the writings of Thomas Hobbes (1588–1679) and John Locke

(1632–1704). John Rawls' original position, discussed in Chapter 2, is a modern version of a social contract approach.

From a consensus perspective, the political process allows different groups to put their views, and laws are made through democratic debate, reflecting wider social values. Admittedly it is possible for the government of the day to pass legislation that is oppressive, unpopular or does not seem to be in the national interest, but in that case they run the risk of being voted out of power at the next election. Legal powers enable the government to ensure that its laws and policies are implemented effectively, but law also limits what it can do and ensures fairness. Governments and government officers must not break the law, and can be held to account if they do. The court acts as a neutral forum to hear cases and appeals, adjudicate on issues and review government decision-making. Consensus approaches do not claim that society is perfect and that there is no need for change, but rather that the system allows for change to happen peacefully. From this viewpoint, legal rights and entitlements can be a powerful force for social change, but it is a reformist approach rather than a radical one.

Furthermore, from a consensus point of view even law's 'failures' have a useful function in society (Durkheim, 1895). Crimes, re-offending, child abuse tragedies and so on cause harm to individuals and society, but paradoxically also serve various purposes for social well-being. Three stand out. First, at a practical level, they create jobs for many people (police, probation and prison officers, lawyers, social workers). Second, they strengthen the bonds between the majority of people, who unite in deploring the events. In this way they assist law's role in social control. And third, strange as it may sound, a certain level of crime is a sign of a healthy society. A society which had no crime at all would be overly repressive, with no room for individual freedom and initiative. Law-breaking has an important role in demonstrating a satisfactory balance between freedom and social control. These three reasons mean that a society with no crime is impossible, not because people are inherently wicked, but because society *needs* crime. Even if all the current crimes were prevented, new offences would be created to fill the gaps.

Conflict (or critical) approaches hold that law serves the interests of the privileged under a mask of fairness for all and equal freedoms for all. Parliamentary democracy and the neutrality of the court disguise the fact that some social groups have much more power and influence than others, much more real freedom to do what they want, not just a formal equality or freedom. Law generally works in their interests, to safeguard their wealth and privilege. We can see this power at work when a law is passed despite strong criticisms from professional experts, or despite widespread public protests. Most of the time, though, we don't see power at work in this overt way. It operates much more quietly, and because of that much more powerfully, through the socialising influences of families, communities, the education system, the mass media and welfare agencies. These social structures shape people's expectations, preventing most cases from ever reaching the formal legal system. The 'little person' doesn't usually get to make their claim and the powerful don't get taken to court. And even if they do, we know that people who can afford good lawyers are more likely to get a favourable decision than those who cannot. We all know the old saying that there's one law for the rich and another for the poor.

There are different branches of critical theory about the law. The major line of thinking is rooted in the writings of Karl Marx, which as we saw earlier highlights the inequities of wealth and ownership, but there are also feminist and anti-racist approaches, and approaches that emphasise the way law stereotypes and disempowers people because of disability, age and sexuality (for overviews, see Wacks, 2009; Travers, 2010).

Conflict models are sceptical about legal rights and the possibilities of social reform via the law. For example, human rights are mistrusted for being individualistic, serving the interests of powerful individuals by preserving their property, status and liberty to accumulate more wealth. Any gains for poorer individuals (or women, black people, disabled people, older people, gay people) are often incidental and relatively unimportant – not to the individuals concerned, certainly, but in terms of wider social inequality. Civil partnerships for gay and lesbian couples might be seen as an example of that. Nothing much has changed about the overall structure of society and the overall balance of power, so in that sense the changes are relatively easily conceded by those at the top. Even so, the ground is rarely given up without a battle, and even small changes often have to be fought for.

Consensus and conflict in practice

There are overlaps as well as differences between the consensus and conflict models. Consensus approaches emphasise the ways that the law can be used to protect individuals, challenge injustice and promote social reform. Conflict theorists have more misgivings about the effectiveness of the law to achieve real change, but are still likely to use it (although they would not rely on it). They would use it because small gains are still gains, and many small gains can eventually bring big change. All changes have to be fought for, and court action and campaigns to change the law are the main routes available to radicals and reformists alike. After that, the law has to be implemented. Conflict perspectives are very wary of the ways that the policies of welfare agencies and the actions of welfare professionals can water down and even distort the potential impact of reformist legislation (McLaughlin, 2005; Preston-Shoot, 2010, 2011). Consensus approaches tend to be more optimistic, but they also accept that legislation is not always put into practice as intended.

Another dimension to the consensus–conflict pairing is that although the courts are often seen as adversarial settings where the different parties fight out their case, in practice the opposing parties very often reach agreement outside the court. This has been described as 'bargaining in the shadow of the law' (Mnookin and Kornhauser, 1979; and see Galanter, 1974). Lawyers very often advise their clients to agree certain matters, or at least not to contest them, or to reduce their demands so that it is easier for the other side to accept them (Parsons, 1954). These techniques are especially well-known in divorce cases (e.g. Eekelaar *et al.*, 2000). There are some pragmatic advantages to this, for lawyers and the courts, because they simply do not have the time to take every case to a full contest; and also, there can be benefits to the clients in honest advice about their chances of success. But there is also concern that out-of-court agreements can too easily be to the advantage of the more powerful party, that the appearance of agreement masks control and coercion. The rights of the socially weaker party must be carefully guarded in negotiations and processes such as mediation and 'alternative dispute resolution' (ADR).

In summary, consensus and conflict understandings differ about whose interests law serves, the whole of society or just the powerful (however they are defined), but both are ready to use the law to promote citizens' and service users' rights. At the practice level, conflict and consensus-seeking approaches interweave all the time, in strategies of bargaining and reaching agreements. In these senses it is not a simple matter of 'either-or', but another 'both-and' pairing, like the four that we discussed in Chapter

1. Law can help to promote social change and social well-being, but the driving force has to come from elsewhere. Law can also individualise people's problems and preserve the *status quo*. The same can be said about social work. It is important to remember both sides of the coin.

Chapter 1

Conclusion

This chapter has explored four dimensions of freedom and two questions about the role of law in society – whether it has the primary role or a secondary role in creating and upholding social values and social order, and whether it works for the good of all or the benefit of the few. The answers to the last question give us a final key pairing for thinking about law, ethics and social work – conflict and consensus.

The chapter has elaborated on themes discussed in the previous chapters, and brought the first part of the book to a close. Part II of the book goes on to apply the concepts and principles to current social work legislation, policy and practice, and leading court cases.

Questions for reflection

- How far should you allow for cultural relativism with regard to:

  a) the age of consent for having sex?

  b) corporal punishment of children?

  c) the clothes that women are expected to wear?

- Do you lean more towards a consensus or conflict understanding of the law and society? What do you base that on? What do you think the implications are for social work?

Useful websites and further reading

The websites and books referred to at the end of previous chapters are useful again to pursue the themes of this chapter.

Bingham (2010) *The Rule of Law*, is a clear and compelling discussion of the importance of law, from the perspective of a former leading judge (now deceased).

For academic overviews of the role of law in society, see:

- Travers (2010) *Understanding Law and Society.*

- Wacks (2009) *Understanding Jurisprudence: An Introduction to Legal Theory.*

Clark (2000) *Social Work Ethics: Politics, Principles and Practice*, is still a useful book for highlighting the social, legal and political contexts of social work ethics.

Summary of Part I

Before moving on to explore how the legal and ethical frameworks apply to social work and real life cases, let's remind ourselves of the core components of our models for thinking about the relationships between social work, law and ethics. In Part I we have identified a range of principles and approaches. There are four key pairings in Chapter 1, and another two added after that; four approaches to fairness, four principles of decision-making, four major ethical schools, and four approaches to freedom.

The key pairings are rights and responsibilities, freedom and control, individual and society, certainty and uncertainty, reason and emotion, and consensus and conflict.

The approaches to fairness in Chapter 2 are justice, equality, human rights and care. Each has two sides: formal and social justice; equality of opportunity and equality of outcome; civil and political rights, and economic, social and cultural rights; the ethical duty of care and the legal duty of care.

The decision-making principles in Chapter 3 are legality, fairness, rationality and proportionality.

The major ethical approaches in Chapter 4 are Kantianism, utilitarianism, virtue ethics and care ethics – in a catchphrase, 'the four Cs': categorical, consequentialist, character and care.

The main approaches to freedom in Chapter 5 are libertarian, radical, relativist and existentialist.

The overlaps and tensions between these elements are crucial to social order and social living, and at the heart of social work. The important message is to try to keep them all in play, to use the strengths of one set of ideas to counteract the limitations of another, to maintain a continual dialogue between them. This dynamic approach gives a basis for creative, fair and caring responses to some of life's most difficult situations.

Part II   Questions and cases

6 End of life decisions

Who can decide when and how someone should die?

Decisions about end of life care and dying raise fundamental questions about the value of human life, individual choice, professionals' opinions and courts' powers. This chapter examines the issues by discussing two types of case – the withdrawal of life-sustaining treatment from a seriously disabled infant, and cases of assisted suicide. The theme of choices, risks and best interests is continued in the next chapter, which discusses the dilemmas that arise when people have limited abilities to understand the consequences of their own decisions.

'Life or death' issues are often in the background, and sometimes the foreground, of social work decision-making. They will be familiar to social workers who work in hospitals or palliative care teams (Beresford et al., 2007; Reith and Payne, 2009). Social workers in other settings are also likely to come across them, at least from time to time, particularly those working with older people and mentally ill people, disabled children and adults, or children at risk of significant harm. When it comes to decisions about withdrawing treatment or assisted suicide, the people involved are likely to be users (or potential users) of social work services (people with disabilities, for example), and relatives under great stress who want the best for the person they love. Crucially, the important issues of choice, best interests and the powers and duties of the state are at the heart of all social work. The end of life angle is an extreme case that helps to expose some of the dilemmas of everyday social work practice.

Life-sustaining treatment

The law requires doctors to preserve the life of their patients, but this does not take precedence over all other considerations. They are not allowed to act with the primary intention of ending a person's life, even out of compassion, but there are times when their task is to ensure that people end their lives with dignity and as comfortably as possible. The principles that doctors have to follow are summarised in guidance from the General Medical Council (GMC, 2010).

There is no obligation to give treatment that is futile or burdensome, and treatment may be withheld or withdrawn if it is not considered clinically appropriate or in the patient's best interests. Assessing a patient's best interests involves weighing up the *benefits, burdens and risks* of further treatment (GMC, 2010). As far as practicable, such decisions should be made in consultation with the patient, colleagues providing care and if relevant with the person's family or nominated representative. There should be the opportunity for people to ask for a second opinion, or seek legal advice if they disagree, but the GMC guidance is to try to get people to talk about the issues, to reach consensus. If agreement is reached, there would not normally have to be a court hearing about it.

The principles and requirements of the Mental Capacity Act 2005 and the related Code of Practice (DCA, 2007a) apply when patients do not have capacity to reach decisions themselves. Mental capacity is discussed in more detail in Chapter 7.

A patient may refuse life-saving treatment, and if they are an adult with the mental capacity to make that decision, it must be respected. People without capacity may have given an 'advance decision' about refusing certain forms of treatment, and if this is considered valid and applicable it must be respected (ss. 24-6 of the Mental Capacity Act 2005). Advance decisions to refuse life-sustaining treatment must be in writing, specify the type of treatment and that the refusal applies even if life is at risk, and must be signed and witnessed. (Doctors *must* apply to court for authorisation to withhold life-sustaining treatment from patients in a vegetative state, or a minimally conscious state, if there is no advance decision: Court of Protection Practice Direction 9E paragraph 5; see *W v M and Others* [2011].)

In the case of an infant or child who lacks competence, it is the parents or others with parental responsibility who should normally make the decision, in consultation with the doctors. (See Chapter 7 for a discussion of 'Gillick competence', and whether the young person can make the decision themselves.) If there is a disagreement or uncertainty either of the parties (the doctors or the parents) may apply to the High Court, for it to decide the matter. The court will make its decision according to its assessment of the child's best interests.

The phrase 'best interests' takes us to the legal and ethical heart of the matter. Let us look at a real case to explore some of the issues in more depth.

When might it be right to allow a child to die?

Before reading further, take time to think about your answer to this question. Who should decide, and how? What are the key factors to consider? What are your initial views? Do they change as you think about it some more?

Box 6.1: Baby RB (2009)

This case involved a baby boy, referred to in the courts as 'RB', who was born in October 2008. The case was heard in the High Court in November 2009, when he was just over a year old (*RB (A Child)* [2009]). In the end the parents reached agreement about what should happen so the judge did not make a final judgment, but did give some 'words of endorsement' to their decision. You can read them on the BAILII website (www.bailii.org.uk). They are very moving. In terms of our reason–emotion pairing, they are carefully reasoned comments, as one would expect from a senior judge, but it would be quite wrong to say that there is no emotion or care in them (for other information about the case, see Day, 2009).

RB was born to a young couple in their twenties, and it was clear from shortly after his birth that he was very seriously disabled. He was diagnosed with a condition called congenital myasthenic syndrome (CMS), which prevents the effective transmission of messages from the brain to the muscles. Apart from being able to make small movements of his lower arms and hands, RB had little control over his limbs. He was never able to breathe without the aid of a ventilation machine, and had to be fed through a tube into his nostril. He could not have survived without continuous and invasive medical treatment, and was never able to leave the special care unit at the hospital.

RB's parents were described as 'exemplary' in their actions towards him, even though their own relationship ended during the course of the year. They spent long periods of time at his bedside, each and every day, doing what they could to care for him and stimulate him. After a year, though, the doctors and his mother agreed that the treatment needed to keep RB alive was causing him such pain and distress that it would be best to turn off the ventilator, knowing that this would lead to his death. His father disagreed. He argued that RB's brain was not affected by the condition, and that with suitable treatment he could have a good quality of life. He wanted RB to have an operation to allow more air to get into his lungs, so that he could go home with a portable ventilation unit. The doctors' opinion was that this would risk more complications and more medical procedures, and bring more pain. The matter came to the High Court, for a hearing that lasted over a week. On the last day, the father changed his mind and agreed that the ventilator should be switched off.

Reading the judge's comments and the newspaper reports of the time, it is very hard to think the decision was wrong. Yet without criticising anyone involved in the case, there are grounds to stop and think about the implications. It is a 'tip of the iceberg' case, in two senses. One is that most cases like this do not come to court at all, because the parents and the doctors agree. This case brings submerged practices to light, so it is worth thinking about. Without any reflection on the people involved in this particular case, we know that patients' rights are not always well-served in medical settings, especially disabled people (e.g. Mencap, 2007, 2102; Michael, 2008; JCHR, 2008). Read and Clements (2004) argue that court cases about withdrawing treatment to disabled children are litmus tests of attitudes towards disabled people more generally.

Second, the case makes us think about 'slippery slope' arguments. If we allow this child to die, what about another, who is nearly as severely disabled, but not quite? Perhaps it would be in that child's best interests to be allowed to die too. And if so, then what about another who is nearly as severely disabled as them, but not quite? And if them, what about the next one, and so on? Where is the cut-off point?

Choosing between healthy babies who are allowed to live and unhealthy ones who are left to die, takes us into some of the most frightening visions of a society that is oppressive and discriminatory. On the other hand, keeping people alive who are in continuing and great pain, when there is no prospect of relief or recovery, only continuing suffering (or people who are 'brain dead', in a vegetative state) – this is an equally frightening picture, just as much a society where rules reign over care and responsiveness to individual circumstances. But any decision to end treatment must be based on a careful assessment of the whole case and the patient's best interests.

The courts take a wide view of the patient's best interests. It is not just about the medical issues, but includes emotional and welfare matters. There is a strong presumption in favour of prolonging life, but this can be rebutted. The court has to weigh up all the factors. This includes the person's wishes and beliefs (or their assumed point of view), but without a valid and applicable advance decision these are not the determinative factor. The assessment must consider the levels of pain and suffering that the treatment may cause, and the likely consequences for their life after the treatment. No assumptions must be made about a person's quality of life, for example on the basis on their age or disability. For a full discussion of the best interests test for children, see the judgment in *Wyatt and Another v Portsmouth NHS Trust and Another* [2005].

Do the approaches in Chapters 4 and 5 shed any light on the case? They do not give us any easy answers, but they do give us a set of frameworks for evaluating the issues. Categorical approaches place high value on human life because of the principle of treating individuals as ends in themselves. The instinct would be to prolong life. However, keeping the child alive in this case, in pain and with no hope of improvement, seems contrary to his individual dignity. So it could be argued from a categorical point of view that withdrawing treatment is consistent with treating him as an end in himself. A utilitarian approach would weigh up the consequences of prolonging the child's life, in terms of the balance of pleasure and pain. On this basis the utilitarian instinct is likely to support the decision to withdraw treatment. However, thinking about it some more, the utilitarian balance sheet is not just

Chapters 4 & 5

about the individual child's happiness or discomfort. What about the wishes of the adults involved, and the wider consequences of this decision for social attitudes towards the care of disabled children? These also have to be taken into the calculation, so on reflection utilitarians may have more reservations about the decision than at first sight.

Looking at the case from the perspective of virtue ethics, the idea of good character puts the emphasis on the parents, to find a middle way between dedicated love and a blind love that does not see the costs to the child. It is a hard task – the mid-point is hard to define and hard to achieve. From a care perspective, the relationships are all important. The parents' care and love for the child was commended by the court; but the ethical challenge might be, out of care and love, to let the child go.

The libertarian approach insists that there must be compelling grounds for the state to intervene in a private, family matter. The focus would be the legitimacy of the intervention, rather than the decision itself. The libertarian position is likely to split between its right and left wing versions. The more conservative side would set great store by the rights of the parents, and require strong evidence of the need to overrule them. In the case of RB, of course, the fact that the parents disagreed was why it came to court. In the end, when the father agreed with the doctors and the mother, the court respected this decision and did not make a judgment. Other libertarians may set greater store by the child's rights, but it would still be a high threshold before the state could impose a solution.

The radical and relativist positions raise some intriguing issues, even if not directly relevant to this particular case. A radical perspective might stress the importance of adequate funding, through general taxation, to support high-quality medical and social care services. It would be sceptical about approaches that reduce the issues to the choices of individuals (whether for or against preserving life), if there are inadequate services to support carers. It would also draw attention to the fact that disability and ill health are not evenly distributed across the social classes. Families with disabled children are more likely to be in the poorer socio-economic groups (Blackburn *et al.*, 2010; Children's Society, 2011), which has implications for the provision of health care and support services. The relativists would draw attention to the social significance of having a disabled child in different cultural groups. For some, it carries considerable stigma and shame. To help the parents, we need to be mindful of the cultural context.

Finally, the existentialist position rejects imposed rules and external truths. Truth comes from within, from acting freely, authentically, and taking responsibility for one's own actions. It is a demanding and personal message, and one might not expect to find it reflected in the court. However, it is useful even here because it reminds us of the importance of listening to the parents, avoiding predefined answers, of being open to understand their positions as individuals and in their social context. An existentialist perspective takes us back to one of our key pairings, certainty and uncertainty. However much we recognise the complexity of the situation, a decision had to be made. The case was brought to court to get certainty. In the end, the father changed his mind. He did not leave it up to the court to decide, but took the responsibility himself, and the judge acknowledged that. Even so, one has to wonder whether this was a genuine, full agreement or more of an acceptance of the inevitable (so in that sense,

Chapter 5

perhaps the apparent consensus masked on-going conflict, the key pairing discussed in Chapter 5). Furthermore, the 'certainty' at the end of court proceedings is never really the end of things. Baby RB died, but his parents have to live with the experiences, and we do not know how that will work out over the years; and the outcome may influence decisions in other cases, again in ways that no-one can predict for sure. The future is never certain.

Assisted dying

There is a great difference between the way that the law and the courts deal with withdrawals or refusals of life-sustaining treatment, cases of euthanasia ('mercy killing'), and cases of assisted suicide. A mentally competent adult is able to refuse life-sustaining treatment, and in law that decision should be respected, even though it will lead to their death. But euthanasia and assisting suicide are both illegal, even if the person concerned is mentally competent and has asked for them, and even if they have a very limited and painful lifespan ahead of them. The phrase 'assisted dying' is sometimes used as an umbrella term to cover both (Bazalgette and Bradley, 2010).

Euthanasia is when someone takes a deliberate action to bring another person's life to an end, such as giving a lethal injection or suffocating them. There is a further distinction to be drawn between voluntary euthanasia (at the person's request) and involuntary. Someone who intentionally ends the life of another, even if the person has asked and the motive is compassionate, is likely to be charged with murder. If they are found guilty, the mandatory sentence is life imprisonment, although in reality this rarely means the rest of the person's life. The judge decides the minimum term that has to be served.

Assisted suicide is when someone helps another person to end their own life, for example by making arrangements for them to self-administer a lethal dose of drugs. Suicide itself is not against the law in the United Kingdom, but assisting someone to commit suicide is (under s. 2 of the Suicide Act 1961), with a possible sentence of up to fourteen years' imprisonment. However, it is not automatic that the person will be prosecuted, and the consent of the Director of Public Prosecutions (DPP) is required before prosecution proceeds. In 2010, the DPP issued guidelines on the factors that would be taken into account in deciding whether or not to prosecute in such cases. It is important to be clear that these apply to assisted suicide only, not to euthanasia. The factors are summarised in Box 6.2.

Assisted suicide: two key cases

Two cases stand out as crucial in changing the approach to assisted suicide, those of Dianne Pretty and Debbie Purdy.

Dianne Pretty was diagnosed with motor neurone disease in November 1999 (note: the court judgments use 'Dianne', but much of the reporting about her case used 'Diane'). This is a degenerative condition which weakens the muscles and eventually leads to death because the person can no longer breathe. Mrs Pretty's physical condition deteriorated quickly, but her intellectual abilities were not affected. She wanted control over when and how she died, and thought that when the time came she might ask her husband to assist her to commit suicide. In July 2001 her solicitors wrote to the DPP on her behalf, asking for an assurance that her husband would not be prosecuted for helping her to commit suicide in accordance with her own wishes. The DPP would not give such an undertaking. Mrs Pretty applied for judicial review of the matter, and her case was heard in the High Court in October 2001.

Mrs Pretty's argument was that the DPP should be required to give the assurance, and that s. 2 of the Suicide Act 1961 was incompatible with Articles 2, 3, 8, 9 and 14 of the European Convention. The High Court rejected her case, and she appealed to the House of Lords (she was allowed to leapfrog the Court of Appeal because of the seriousness and urgency of the matter). They heard the case in November 2001, and also rejected it (*R (Pretty) v Director of Public Prosecutions* [2001]). They did not agree that the right to life (Article 2) included a right to die, or that the right not to suffer inhuman and degrading treatment (Article 3) created a duty on the state to allow her to die. The House of Lords did not accept that the Article 8 rights to private and family life were even engaged, holding that they did not extend to the right to decide when and how to die. Mrs Pretty's claims about Article 9, freedom of conscience, and Article 14, freedom from discrimination, were also rejected. Mrs Pretty then took her case to the European Court of Human Rights, where it was heard in April 2002 (*Pretty v United Kingdom* [2002]). Again, her case was rejected, but the European Court did hold that her Article 8 rights were involved, because her choice about the manner of her dying was part of her life. However, it concluded that s. 2 of the Suicide Act was a legitimate and proportionate interference with this right in order to protect vulnerable people from being exploited. Mrs Pretty died in a hospice less than two weeks after the judgment.

Press coverage of Mrs Pretty's case tended to be sympathetic to her, as indeed were the court judgments, even when refusing her application. She came across as a determined woman, fighting for what she wanted. But the disability rights campaigner Baroness Jane Campbell gives a different view. In a powerfully written chapter, she contends:

> Diane Pretty was presented to the press as a tragic and pathetic individual. She received maximum coverage, none of which questioned, even fleetingly, her suicidal tendencies ... Against this backdrop the general public could be forgiven for believing that anyone with a substantial level of disability will inevitably be deeply depressed and preoccupied with thoughts of dying ... I never met Diane but I wish we could have spent some time together. Her life was very different from mine and I would have liked to know the reasons for that. Did she choose to live in a downstairs room rather than have adaptations to her home or be rehoused? Did she want her husband to be a full time carer rather than accept more support from social services? ... Epithets such as 'tragic', 'burdensome' and even 'desperate' are frequently used to describe disabled people's lives, and unless you are extraordinarily strong it's all too easy for disabled people to succumb to this negativity and internalize this oppression which could end in their suicide.
>
> (Campbell, 2008: 91)

It is a challenging viewpoint, although it seems unlikely that no-one had tried to have those discussions with Mrs Pretty. The court accepted that she was competent to make her decision and was doing so of her free will. But Campbell's argument is important because it reflects a very different approach to disability, a social perspective rather than a narrowly medical or legal one. With adequate services and a more positive social environment, perhaps there would be no reason for someone to consider an assisted death.

The second key case is that of Debbie Purdy. There are some similarities with Dianne Pretty's case, but a different outcome. Ms Purdy was diagnosed with multiple sclerosis in 1995, another degenerative and currently incurable condition. By 2007 the condition was advanced. In December 2007, her solicitors wrote to the DPP on her behalf, asking him to publish any guidelines he might have about whether or not to prosecute someone for assisting suicide (and if he did not have any, to make them). This was because Ms Purdy wanted to be sure that her husband would not be prosecuted if he assisted her to travel abroad to commit suicide. If she could not be sure about this, then she would have to travel sooner rather than later, while she could still do it without his help. Her argument was that knowing the principles would enable them to reach an informed decision, and would mean that she could live longer than if she had to second guess what would happen.

The DPP replied in January 2008, saying that there was no such policy. In April 2008 Ms Purdy made a claim for judicial review. The High Court and then the Court of Appeal both rejected her claim. However, the ground was shifting because between those two hearings, in December 2008, the DPP published his reasons for deciding not to prosecute the parents and a friend of Daniel James, a young man who had been paralysed as a result of a rugby accident. He had been determined to commit suicide, and although his parents had tried hard to convince him not to, in the end they had assisted him to go to Switzerland, where the organisation Dignitas helps terminally ill people to die. They were not prosecuted.

Ms Purdy's case was heard by the House of Lords in June 2009 (*R (Purdy v Director of Public Prosecutions [2009]*). It held that the Article 8 right to private life was engaged in this case. The consequence is that any interference by the state must be legal and proportionate, and the reasons for it must be transparent. For this reason, the decision was that the DPP should publish guidelines about the factors to be taken into account. Interim guidelines were published in September 2009 and the final version in February 2010.

One of the key features is the importance of the suspect's motive (the guidelines acknowledge that the terms 'suspect' and 'victim' can seem awkward). Characteristics of the victim, such as being old or disabled, do not justify not prosecuting. A controversial element is that if the suspect is involved with the victim in a professional role, this makes it more likely they will be charged. The campaign group Dignity in Dying (discussed further below) argues this leaves assisted suicide as an amateur matter, and offers less assurance to people that matters will be well handled.

> **Box 6.2: Guidelines on prosecuting cases of encouraging or assisting suicide (DPP, 2010)**
>
> The guidelines from the Director of Public Prosecutions list 18 factors which would point towards prosecution (para. 43). These include if the victim is under 18 years of age; the victim did not have the capacity (under the Mental Capacity Act 2005) to reach an informed decision; the suspect was not wholly motivated by compassion (but, for example, by the prospect of gain); the suspect pressured the victim into committing suicide; the suspect was acting in a professional capacity and the victim was in their care.
>
> Paragraph 45 states:
>
> > A prosecution is less likely to be required if:
> >
> > 1   the victim had reached a voluntary, clear, settled and informed decision to commit suicide;
> >
> > 2   the suspect was wholly motivated by compassion;
> >
> > 3   the actions of the suspect, although sufficient to come within the definition of the offence, were of only minor encouragement or assistance;
> >
> > 4   the suspect had sought to dissuade the victim from taking the course of action which resulted in his or her suicide;
> >
> > 5   the actions of the suspect may be characterised as reluctant encouragement or assistance in the face of a determined wish on the part of the victim to commit suicide;
> >
> > 6   the suspect reported the victim's suicide to the police and fully assisted them in their enquiries into the circumstances of the suicide or the attempt and his or her part in providing encouragement or assistance.

The on-going debate

The law, principles and circumstances under which a person may be assisted to die, or have life-sustaining treatment withdrawn, remain highly controversial. There is regular media coverage of cases involving difficult end of life decisions – where people wish for help to die, or where people have taken matters into their own hands and ended the life of a relative or friend, or where the court has made decisions about whether or not to withdraw treatment. There was a prominent example of the latter in 2011, when the Court of Protection ruled against withdrawing life-sustaining treatment for a patient in a state of minimal consciousness (*W v M and Others* [2011]). (In this case, the judge concluded his

Chapter 12

judgment by saying that cases of this sort should be reported as widely and freely as possible, provided that the privacy of the individuals is respected, to raise public understanding of the issues. The question of media reporting of court cases is discussed further in Chapter 12.)

There have been attempts in England and Scotland to introduce legislation to allow assisted dying in specified circumstances and with careful safeguards. These have been rejected in both countries. In England, the Assisted Dying for the Terminally Ill Bill was voted down by the House of Lords in May 2006, and in Scotland, the End of Life Assistance (Scotland) Bill was rejected in November 2010.

An organisation that argues for assisted dying is Dignity in Dying, which was formerly known as the Voluntary Euthanasia Society. They use the term assisted dying in a specific way, not as an umbrella term but specifically for people who are terminally ill. They argue that there should be good quality care for people at the end of their lives, but that mentally competent adults who are terminally ill should have the choice of an assisted death. They reject slippery slope arguments, saying that there is no evidence of this in places that do allow assisted dying, such as the Netherlands and Oregon in the USA (Dignity in Dying, 2006: 19).

An organisation that argues against them is Care Not Killing, a UK-based alliance of groups that wish to promote better end of life care and are opposed to all forms of euthanasia, assisted suicide and assisted dying. One of their principal objections is that older and disabled people will be seen as less worthy of proper care and support if there is a weakening of the law. It will undermine their rights and place them at risk of having their lives ended, when they could have received treatment and support to continue living well (also Campbell's argument, 2008). For opponents of assisted dying, the right to life is fundamental and the wider interests of society (to protect this right for all) outweigh individual choice.

In November 2010, Dignity in Dying helped to set up a Commission on Assisted Dying. The briefing paper for the Commission by Bazalgette and Bradley (2010) is a useful summary of research and of differences in legislation and practice between different countries, and well worth reading. The Commission was hosted by the think-tank Demos. It described itself as independent, but Care Not Killing did not believe that it was and refused to cooperate with it. The Commission took evidence during 2011, and published its report in January 2012 (CAD, 2012).

The report argues that assisted dying should be lawful for people who are terminally ill, by which they mean a life expectancy of less than 12 months. They must be adults with mental capacity, making a truly voluntary and informed choice. The patient must take the final action to end their own life. The Commission proposes various safeguards, such as needing independent opinions from two doctors, and training and a code of practice for health and social care professionals involved. They also call for improvements in end of life care.

Conclusion

This chapter has discussed the questions of when it might be right to withdraw life-sustaining treatment from a disabled child, and whether it should be lawful to assist a mentally competent adult to commit suicide if they have clearly indicated that this is their wish.

As noted at the start of the chapter, end of life decisions raise dilemmas that are fundamental in social work, about the tensions between individual choice, professional opinion and the powers of the state – what's the right thing to do, what's the good thing to do, what's the legal thing to do? They touch on all the key issues of rights and responsibilities, freedom and choice, the individual and society, certainty and uncertainty. They present challenges for all four ethical schools and the different understandings of freedom. The next chapter adds to the picture by looking at questions of autonomy and choice when the individuals concerned have limited capabilities.

Questions for reflection

- Look back to the quotation from Baroness Campbell, about Dianne Pretty. What do you think? Was Mrs Pretty really the victim of internalised social prejudice against disabled people, or a clear thinking person trying to protect her husband and end her life as she wished?

- Do you think that assisted suicide should be legal? What about euthanasia?

- How do notions of categorical duties, consequences, virtue and care influence your thinking? And what about the different freedoms – from undue state control, from oppression, for cultural respect, and for individuals to be truly authentic?

- What would you say and do if a service user said to you that they were thinking of committing suicide?

Useful websites and further reading

SCIE End of life care hub: www.scie.org.uk/adults/endoflifecare/index.asp

Dignity in Dying: www. dignityindying.org.uk

Compassion in Dying is a charity set up by Dignity in Dying to provide advice and information around rights and choices to people at the end of their lives: www.compassionindying.org.uk

Care Not Killing: www.carenotkilling.org.uk

Commission on Assisted Dying: www.commissiononassisteddying.co.uk

BBC ethics website on euthanasia: www.bbc.co.uk/ethics/euthanasia

Questions and cases

NHS 'National End of Life Care Programme' website: www.endoflifecareforadults.nhs.uk

National End of Life Care Programme (2010) *Supporting People to Live and Die Well: A Framework for Social Care at the End of Life*.

'Together for Short Lives' is a voluntary organisation to represent and help children and families when a child is terminally ill: www.togetherforshortlives.org.uk

General Medical Council (2010) *Treatment and Care Towards the End of Life: Good Practice in Decision-Making*, via the GMC website.

Clements and Read (eds) (2008) *Disabled People and the Right to Life: The Protection and Violation of Disabled People's Most Basic Human Rights*.

7 Choices, capacity and competence

How much freedom do people have to make choices that appear to be against their own best interests?

Freedom is a central principle in ethics and law, as discussed in previous chapters. For social policy and social work, an important aspect of it is empowering people to make choices and take greater control of their own lives. However, this can also bring risks for people, especially those who have limited capacity (for whatever reason) to foresee and understand the likely consequences of their decisions. Sometimes a person's choices may place them in situations where they are at risk of abuse or exploitation, or their choices may be coerced by people who are a danger to them. In other cases the risks are those of everyday living (say, a person with mobility problems living alone, with a risk of falling), or of preferences and pleasures (for example, choices about leisure activities that may carry risks). There are also dilemmas when people make decisions, or want to make decisions, about ending their own lives, as we saw in the previous chapter.

The balancing of choices and risks has always been one of the central challenges for social work, but it has become even more prominent in recent years because of the rise of personalisation as an overarching theme in social policy and public services. The drive is for service users to have greater control over their own lives and the services they receive.

There are two useful 'best practice guides' issued by the Department of Health that offer guidelines and ideas for balancing choices and risks. The first, issued under the Labour government, is *Independence, Choice and Risk: A Guide to Best Practice in Supported Decision-Making* (DH, 2007). It is concerned with how best to help people make everyday choices and decisions. It emphasises the benefits of proportionate risk-taking, but notes that local authorities have a responsibility not to agree a care plan if it seems likely to place an individual in a dangerous situation.

The second key document is *Practical Approaches to Safeguarding and Personalisation* (DH, 2010a), issued under the coalition government. It states that:

> Personalisation is about enabling people to lead the lives that they choose and achieve the outcomes they want in ways that best suit them. It is important in this process to consider risks, and keeping people safe from harm. However, risks need to be weighed alongside benefits. Risk should not be an excuse to restrict people's lives.

(DH, 2010a: 5)

This chapter explores some of the ethical, legal and practical challenges that arise from this approach to choice and managing risks (see also DH, 2009; Carr, 2010). The policy statements are easy to make but can give rise to very difficult dilemmas in practice. This is especially so when there are questions about an adult's mental capacity to truly understand the decision they are making, or a child's competence to do so. The chapter starts by summarising the law that applies in such cases for people aged 16 and over, the Mental Capacity Act 2005. It goes on to discuss a high-profile court case that tested the limits of choice, capacity and consent to sexual relations. Later, it discusses the issue of children's competence to make risky decisions.

Adults' choices and mental capacity

The legal presumption is that mentally competent adults can make their own choices and run their own risks. As we saw in Chapter 6, this is not quite so straightforward if their choices require other people to do something against the law (assist them to commit suicide), even though what they want

Chapter 6

to do is not itself illegal. But what is the position for someone who does not have the level of understanding to make the decision in question, for example because of a learning disability or mental ill-health? The law that applies in such cases in England and Wales is the Mental Capacity Act 2005, summarised in Box 7.1.

Box 7.1: Mental Capacity Act 2005: guiding principles

Notions of legality, fairness, rationality and proportionality provide a general framework for public authorities when making decisions about individual cases and general service provision, as discussed in Chapter 3. There is also a specific framework to guide decision-making for, or on behalf of, individuals who do not have the mental capacity to make the decision in question for themselves. This is the Mental Capacity Act 2005 (MCA), which came into force in 2007. The aim

 was to update and rationalise the law, and give statutory force to principles which had previously been reflected in common law, human rights legislation and good practice (see Brown and Barber, 2008). Section 1 of the Act sets out five guiding principles:

- A person must be assumed to have capacity unless it is established that he lacks capacity.

- A person is not to be treated as unable to make a decision unless all practicable steps to help him to do so have been taken without success.

- A person is not to be treated as unable to make a decision merely because he makes an unwise decision.

- An act done, or decision made, . . . for or on behalf of a person who lacks capacity must be done, or made, in his best interests.

- Before the act is done, or the decision is made, regard must be had to whether the purpose for which it is needed can be as effectively achieved in a way that is less restrictive of the person's rights and freedom of action.

 The Act has two codes of practice: a general one (DCA, 2007a) and a supplementary one dealing with the Deprivation of Liberty Safeguards, 'DOLS' (MoJ, 2008a). These safeguards apply to people in care homes or hospitals, and are discussed further in Chapter 13.

The MCA allows people to plan ahead for the care and treatment they wish to receive should they lose capacity in the future. This includes 'Lasting Powers of Attorney' to deal with their financial affairs and health and welfare matters, and 'advance decisions' about treatment that they do not wish to receive. The Act created the role of Independent Mental Capacity Advocate (IMCA) to represent and support people who lack capacity and who do not have any one else to support them, when a major decision has to be made. It also created the Office of the Public Guardian to protect the interests of people who lack capacity, and a new Court of Protection at High Court level to deal with MCA matters.

The MCA applies to people over 16 who lack capacity because of 'an impairment of, or a disturbance in the functioning of, the mind or brain' (s. 2). Examples are where the individual concerned has dementia, mental health problems or learning disabilities, but it is not limited to those situations. It applies in all cases where a person is mentally incapacitated, whether permanently or temporarily; so, for example, it covers cases where the person lacks capacity because of drug or alcohol misuse, illness or injury. But in all cases there must be an assessment of the person's capacity, no assumption that they cannot decide just because of their disability, illness, age or appearance. The assessment must be linked to the specific decision required (i.e. just because they cannot take one type of decision does not mean they cannot make others). Every effort must be made to help the person understand their choices and make the decision (e.g. waiting until they recover, using sign language, straightforward words or drawings, getting help from family, friends, interpreters or specialist advisers). An unwise or eccentric decision does not mean that the person is incapable, although one would want to assess whether they really understood the consequences of their decision.

If it is necessary for someone else to make the decision, they must do so in the best interests of the person concerned. This involves considering the person's past and present wishes and feelings, and the beliefs and values that would be likely to influence their decision if they had capacity; and the views of relevant family, friends or carers (MCA 2005, s. 4(6)–(7)). Notice though that the decision has to be made in the person's best interests, not necessarily in accordance with their wishes. Further, it is not lawful to deprive someone of their liberty, even if this is considered in their best interests, without proper authorisation (this is either by court order or through the DOLS scheme). Finally, the aim must always be to intervene in the least restrictive way possible, consistent with the person's best interests, and to think creatively about the options for this. One straightforward option is to ask whether the decision really has to be made now, and if not whether the person might be better able to make it at a different time.

The Act gives five vital principles, but McDonald (2010) shows just how hard it can be to put them into practice. Her study of social workers' approaches to assessments under the MCA found that their decision-making was shaped by pressures from other agencies, resource shortages and ambivalent attitudes towards the rights of older people. The challenge for social workers is to make the legislation a reality in all their dealings with all service users. The challenges of balancing choice and safety are well shown in the case of 'MM'.

The case of MM (2007)

The case of *Local Authority X v MM and KM* [2007] was heard in the High Court in June 2007 (hearing *No. 1*), which was before the Mental Capacity Act 2005 was fully implemented and the new Court of Protection established (on 1 October that year). However, the general principles that shaped the MCA were already well established in common law, and guided the court's decisions. The judgment was delivered on 21 August 2007, and there was a review hearing in November 2007 (hearing *No. 2*). The case is also discussed by Laird (2010) and Mandelstam (2011).

MM was 38 years old when the case was heard in summer 2007. She has a learning disability and suffers from paranoid schizophrenia. She had a difficult childhood including sexual abuse by her brother, and was taken into care at the age of 13. She had a long-standing relationship with KM, a man who had been diagnosed with a psychopathic personality disorder and was a heavy alcohol user. He was alleged to have spent her benefit money on alcohol. He had also been violent towards her, and had served a prison sentence for stabbing MM in the leg. He led a nomadic life and encouraged MM to move around with him, and disengage from psychiatric services.

In March 2006, MM moved into supported accommodation. There was an agreement that KM would not attend the unit, but on a number of occasions MM left the unit and stayed away with him. In June 2006 the local authority heard that KM was planning to take MM away to a different part of the country. They applied to court for a declaration that she lacked the capacity to decide where she should live, and an order was made that she should not be removed from the unit. However, she did leave it, and by the time she was found and returned she was in a poor state of health. Her behaviour was aggressive and this put her placement at the unit at risk. In October 2006 she was compulsorily admitted to hospital for assessment under s. 2 of the Mental Health Act 1983. She then went to an adult family placement, but this broke down, and then to a new supported living placement.

When the case came before Mr Justice Munby (now Lord Justice Munby), in June 2007, the local authority sought a number of declarations, including that MM lacked capacity to decide where and with whom she should live, and with whom she should have contact. They did accept that she had capacity to consent to sexual relations. Their plan was that MM should have supervised contact with KM, once per month, for two hours, at a venue to be decided by them. Their concern was that if KM had unsupervised contact with MM, he would say things to her which would undermine the placement. MM and KM opposed the authority's plan. They argued that they wanted to spend time together privately, and under conditions where they could have sexual relations.

Before reading further, take time to think about the key issues in this case. What are the important legal principles, provisions and requirements? What are the ethical issues? Accepting that you only have limited information, what do you think would be the right approach to take, and what are your reasons?

The court had the advantage of more information. There were expert reports from a consultant psychiatrist and an independent social work consultant, and also an assessment from the Official Solicitor, who had been invited to act on MM's behalf. By the end of the hearing, there was an agreement that there should be direct, unsupervised contact between MM and KM, once a week for at least four hours, giving them the opportunity to have sexual relations.

The important legal principle for this case is that mental capacity is *issue-specific*. MM may not have been able to decide where she should live, but she did have an understanding of sex, and her views could not be overridden on the grounds that she did not have capacity to make that decision. It may seem surprising that she was considered not to have capacity to decide about contact, but to have capacity to decide about sex. Having sex with another person requires some form of contact between them. The judge himself admitted that he found this puzzling at first (para. 95 of the judgment). But it returns to the fact that capacity is issue-specific. Contact is a much broader and potentially more complex matter than just understanding about sex. An external observer may or may not think it a wise decision, but that is not the point: MM understood the facts and risks of sexual intercourse well enough to make her own decision. So on that issue she was competent to decide, and therefore the local authority had to consider how it could meet her wishes.

The Mental Capacity Act 2005 is crucial for cases like MM's. Look back to the five guiding principles of the Act in Box 7.1 and consider how they apply to this case. Even on issues where the person is considered *not* to have capacity, the principles still require the least restrictive approach possible to their rights and freedom of action.

Another key legal aspect is Article 8 of the European Convention on Human Rights. This is the right to respect for private and family life. Any interference with this right must be in pursuit of a legitimate aim and proportionate to the risks and matters at stake. Furthermore, the duty to respect private and family life imposes positive duties on a state to uphold and promote it, not merely the duty to abstain from inappropriate interference.

There was a long-standing and strong relationship between MM and KM, which had previously involved sexual relations. Now, the state was interfering with that in the decision about where MM should live; but was it legitimate and proportionate to end all sexual relations between them? Mr Justice Munby decided, very strongly, that it was not. As he expressed it,

> the court must be careful to ensure that in rescuing a vulnerable adult from one type of abuse it does not expose her to the risk of treatment at the hands of the state which, however well intentioned, can itself end up being abusive of her dignity, her happiness and indeed of her human rights.
>
> (*Local Authority X v MM and KM* (No. 1) [2007], para. 118).

A number of ethical perspectives come into play. There is a strong element of utilitarianism in the judgment:

> The emphasis must be on sensible risk appraisal, not striving to avoid all risk, whatever the price, but instead seeking a proper balance . . . in particular to achieve the vital good of the vulnerable person's *happiness*. What good is it making someone safer if it merely makes them miserable?
>
> (*Local Authority X v MM and KM* (No. 1)[2007], para. 120, italics in the original).

Kantians would not be persuaded by the argument about happiness, but they would be convinced by the notion of proportionate interference. People should be treated as ends in themselves, with only the minimum necessary interference with their individuality and autonomy. Aspects of care ethics are reflected in the importance given to the relationship between MM and KM, recognising the affection between them, whatever its flaws. The emphasis on respecting the decisions of an autonomous individual also reflects aspects of libertarianism, relativism and existentialism.

In a more recent case, another judge commented that questions regarding capacity to consent to sexual relations are sensitive and difficult, and a 'legal fog' (*A Local Authority v H* [2012]). In that case, the judge ruled that H (a 29-year-old woman with learning difficulties, autism and a history of highly sexualised behaviour) did not have capacity to consent to sexual relations. This was because she could not understand the health implications, and could not effectively use such knowledge as she did have when she was sexually aroused. He made an order to protect her best interests that he considered very restrictive, amounting to a deprivation of her liberty (para. 1 of the judgment). The judge said that he would review the matter after a year, to see if such restrictions were still necessary. The court had to balance protection and freedom, including people's freedom to make unwise choices. It should only restrict that freedom if and when the best interests of the person positively require so (para. 35).

Children's choices and competence

The law is rather ambivalent about children's rights to make their own choices, and a young person's 'right to die' demonstrates the issues very clearly. Letting children and young people follow their own choices may not always be acceptable to parents, professionals and the courts, if the consequences are likely to be harmful, and especially if there is a risk of the young person's death. It is a good example of the freedom and control pairing in Chapter 1 – there is plenty of rhetoric about free choice, but what happens when people choose the 'wrong' thing?

The starting point for thinking about young people's rights to make their own choices is the notion of 'Gillick competence'. The term comes from the case of *Gillick v West Norfolk and Wisbech Area Health Authority* [1986], discussed in Box 7.2. The case was about consent to receive advice on contraception, but the implications of the judgment go wider than that, establishing important principles for children's autonomy and their rights to make their own decisions, independently of their parents.

Box 7.2: Gillick competence

In 1980, the Department of Health issued guidance to area health authorities about doctors giving contraceptive advice to young people under 16 years of age. It stated that the normal procedure should be to have parental consent, and if at all possible doctors should encourage the young person to involve their parent; but if this was not appropriate, the doctor should go ahead without parental involvement. Mrs Gillick sought an assurance from her health authority that her family GP would not prescribe contraception to her daughters, then aged under 16, without first informing her and obtaining her agreement. The authority could not give that assurance, and Mrs Gillick took the case to court on two grounds – first, that prescribing contraception to young people under 16 amounted to aiding and abetting under-age sex, and second that it undermined her parental rights because (under the Family Law Reform Act 1969), the age at which young people could give consent themselves to medical treatment was 16, not younger.

The case eventually reached the House of Lords (*Gillick v West Norfolk and Wisbech Area Health Authority* [1986]). As regards the first complaint, the decision was that the doctor would not be acting illegally in prescribing contraception if the young person understood the advice and it was in the interests of her own health. The point is that the doctor's motive is safeguard the young person's health, not to encourage under-age sex. The doctor should still try to get the young person to discuss the matter with their parent, but if this could not be achieved, then it would be acceptable to go ahead without parental agreement.

As regards the question of parental rights, the judgment of Lord Scarman has become famous: 'parental rights yield to the child's right to make his own decisions when he reaches a sufficient understanding and intelligence to be capable of making up his own mind on the matter requiring decision.'

The point is that there is no fixed age at which children acquire competence – it depends on their level of understanding and the matter in question. Like mental capacity, it depends on the circumstances. So, for example, a 12-year-old of average ability will be able to make some decisions for themselves, but not others; and a mature and intelligent 12-year-old might well be able to make some decisions that would be too demanding for a less able older child. The concept has become an important principle for children's rights generally, not just medical treatment.

The Gillick judgment was challenged in 2006, when a parent, Sue Axon, applied for judicial review of an up-dated version of the Department of Health guidance about giving contraceptive advice to young people aged under 16 years old (DH, 2004). The case is known as *R (Axon) v Secretary of State for Health (Family Planning Association Intervening)* [2006]. A key factor was that the Human Rights Act had been passed in the meantime, implementing the ECHR in UK law. Ms Axon argued (amongst other things) that her Article 8 rights to private and family life were infringed by the guidance that allowed doctors to give contraceptive advice and treatment to her children without informing her. The judge did not accept that argument, holding (a) that parents had no Article 8 rights over medical advice to a Gillick competent child (although the young person should be encouraged to discuss the matter with their parents); and (b) even if they did, restricting those rights would still be permissible under Article 8(2), which allows for proportionate interference with privacy rights 'for the protection of health or . . . the rights and freedoms of others' (for a commentary on the case, see Taylor, 2007).

Although the Gillick judgment appears to give competent children the right to make their own decisions about medical treatment, the courts swiftly retreated from this position as regards life or death decisions (Douglas, 1992; Taylor, 2007). The idea that children could be considered competent to refuse potentially life-saving treatment seemed too daunting a step to take. One way round it is simply to decide that the young person is not Gillick competent. Fortin (2009: 153–5) observes that the more dangerous the choice, the more likely the courts are to deem the child or young person incompetent. If that is the decision, then a person with parental responsibility would probably be able to decide about treatment, although that would depend on the circumstances of the case, including the age and wishes of the child, the nature of the treatment and the level of force that might have to be used to bring it about. A parent's power to make decisions for their child cannot go beyond what is reasonable, sometimes called the 'zone of parental control' (discussed further below: see DH, 2008b; NIMHE, 2009). If the parent's consent is not considered sufficient, then independent authorisation must be obtained, either under the Mental Health Act 1983 (if the criteria are met) or a court order.

What if the child is refusing life-saving treatment but cannot be declared Gillick incompetent? In the past, the court tried to deal with this predicament by distinguishing between *giving* consent and *refusing* consent. In the case of *Re W (A Minor) (Refusal of Medical Treatment)* [1992], the court held that young people aged 16 or 17, and younger children who were judged to be Gillick competent, were able to give their own consent to medical treatment, but their refusal could be overruled by a person with parental responsibility, or by the court. Indeed, even their consent could be overruled if that was considered in their best interests, but only by the court.

This decision was much criticised by some commentators (for helpful discussions see Fortin, 2006, 2009; Lyons, 2010). Overcoming a refusal might mean having to take quite drastic action to enforce treatment, so is not a step that should be underestimated. Since that judgment, understandings of children's rights and welfare, and of parents' rights and responsibilities, have moved on considerably. It is now most unlikely that the consent of the parent would be seen as enough to warrant medical treatment if a competent child or young person was refusing (discussed further below) (DH, 2008b: paras 36.33–4).

Rights, responsibilities and best interests

The question of children's choices relates to the key tension between rights and responsibilities. Children have rights to express their views, but they do not have a right for those wishes to be fulfilled. The wishes have to be given due consideration in the light of the child's age and understanding (Children Act 1989, s. 1(3)), but the court's paramount consideration is the child's best interests (Children Act 1989, s. 1(1)). The court has to decide according to its view of the child's best interests, not simply in accordance with the child's wishes. (The same principles are in the United Nations Convention on the Rights of the Child, Articles 12 and 3.)

The child's wishes have to be balanced against their other rights, notably to life and development, and to protection from harm. They also have to be balanced against the parents' rights. The Children Act

1989 introduced the notion of 'parental responsibility' which was seen as ending old notions of parents 'owning' their children or having rights to their services. Instead, the emphasis was on their responsibilities to care for and raise their children properly. But the notion of parental rights never went away (it was not abolished but was incorporated in the definition of parental responsibility in s. 3 of the Act,

 discussed further in Chapter 8), and has been reinvigorated by the passing of the Human Rights Act 1998. This makes it clear that parents' rights cannot be overruled without good cause and due process, and that however irresponsible a parent has been, they still have rights to a fair hearing.

At the same time though, as noted earlier, our understanding of children's rights has developed, and it has become even more important to ascertain and respect their wishes. In current legal thinking, it is very unlikely that a parent would be able to overrule a Gillick competent child's refusal of medical treatment. Instead, it might be possible for authorisation to be given under the Mental Health Act, or by the court (depending on the circumstances, applications might be possible under the Mental Capacity Act, the Children Act 1989, or the court's inherent jurisdiction). If the child is not Gillick competent, the consent of the person with parental responsibility will often be sufficient, but as noted above, the specific circumstances may mean that it is not.

The notion that underlies this change of approach is called the 'zone of parental control', described in chapter 36 of the 2008 revised Mental Health Act Code of Practice (DH, 2008b; see also NIMHE, 2009; Bowers and Dubicka, 2009). Although this part of the Code is specifically about the treatment of children and young people with mental health problems, the principles have wider implications. The question is, what sort of decisions can properly be made by parents on behalf of their children, without further scrutiny and authorisation? There are three main areas to be considered when deciding if a decision falls within the zone of parental control:

* What is the nature of the decision? Is it one that a parent would normally be expected to make, bearing in mind general social standards and human rights considerations? Factors to be considered are the invasiveness of the treatment, the strength of any resistance and the age and maturity of the child. The nature of the treatment alone may be enough to take the case beyond the zone of parental control, if it is particularly invasive.

* Are there any indications that the parent may not be acting in the best interests of the child?

* Does the parent have the mental capacity to make the decision in question?

If it appears that a decision might fall outside the zone of parental control, then other authorisation might have to be sought. The term is relatively new and unfamiliar in England. It comes from ECtHR judgments, and does not feature in English law. It is in the Code of Practice for England, but not in the Welsh version. The Code for Wales captures the notion with the simple sentence that the assistance of the court may be necessary 'if a person with parental responsibility is thought not to be acting in the best interests of the child, or if the matter is considered to be outside their responsibility as parent' (WAG, 2008: 210). The zone of parental control has been described as an 'elusive' concept (Barber *et al.* 2012: 141), but what is clear (and very familiar) is that parents do not have absolute control over their children. Rather, parental rights, powers and duties are limited by the child's best interests, wider social standards about proper parenting and the growing independence of the child.

A young person's choice to refuse medical treatment

> **Box 7.3: A teenager's choice**
>
> Imagine that you are the social worker for a family with a 13-year-old girl who has a long history of poor health because of a heart condition. She is an intelligent and thoughtful young woman. She is very unwell at the moment and doctors consider that she needs a heart transplant. The girl is refusing this, saying that she is worn out with the long and painful struggle, with never being able to take part in regular activities and family life, with always feeling sick, with the never-ending tests and treatments. Her parents love her very much and do not want to lose her, but they do not want to force treatment on her or cause her extra pain.
>
> - What are the ethical issues at stake? Consider the four major ethical approaches and the four approaches to freedom.
>
> - What are the legal issues? (Review the material above to help you answer this.)
>
> - What do you think should happen? How do you decide?

Situations where children are dying are very distressing, but Kantian and utilitarian perspectives alike require us to try to put emotion to one side and be rational about what to do (the reason–emotion pairing). Even so, neither of them gives a straightforward answer. Kantians set the highest value on individual human life, treating people as ends not only as means – so that would make it important to keep her alive. But if the young person is competent and her express wish is to be allowed to die, would it not be more respectful of her as an autonomous individual to allow that? From a utilitarian point of view, allowing the girl to die would end her pain, but cause great pain to her parents. Does her parents' happiness outweigh hers? Utilitarians also weigh up the wider social implications: would it be better for society as a whole if young people in this situation were allowed to choose to die, or would it be a happier society in the long run if their wishes were overruled? Do virtue or care ethics add anything? What would the good person do, or the truly caring parent?

The case study in Box 7.3 is based on a real life case from England, that of a 13-year-old girl called Hannah Jones (Jones and Jones, 2010). This hit the news in November 2008 (Barkham, 2008). Doctors had recommended a heart transplant, but Hannah said she did not want this. She had been in and out of hospital since she was diagnosed with leukaemia when she was 4. Her parents and the doctors treating her accepted her choice, but then, after a different doctor had seen her, the health trust made a court application to order treatment. Later, after Hannah and her parents had been interviewed by a specialist nurse, they withdrew the application. Some months later, in summer 2009, Hannah changed her mind and agreed to a transplant.

Hannah's story contrasts with a similar case in 1999, that of a 15-year-old girl who said she did not want to undergo a heart transplant (*Re M (child: refusal of medical treatment)* [1999]). In that case the judge ordered that the operation should go ahead. (The case is some time ago now, and before the Human Rights Act 1998 was implemented.) A key difference is that M had become ill very quickly, unlike Hannah who had been unwell for a very long time. The account of *M*'s views in the judgment shows her state of confusion, whereas Hannah seems to have had a clearer and more consistent understanding. Also, the situation was more urgent in M's case, and she was not expected to live long at all without the transplant. Although Hannah's life expectancy was poor, it was not an emergency. It is also important to know that after the judge ordered the operation, M changed her mind and agreed to it.

If the ultimate goal was to keep the young people alive, we could say that in the end both M and Hannah's cases reached the right result – but one by overruling the child's wishes, the other by respecting them. In both cases, the young people eventually agreed to the treatment, but it was not certain that they would. Hannah's parents would have chosen for her to have the operation, but above all wanted to back her decision (Jones and Jones, 2010: 291). In such difficult situations, what is important is that the individuals concerned can give a reasoned and caring account of why they reached the decision they did.

Conclusion

This chapter has explored the realities and dilemmas of upholding people's rights to choose, when they are vulnerable (in the examples discussed, by reason of learning disability and young age), and those choices place them at risk. The chapter has introduced the crucial concepts of capacity and competence. For adults, the assumption is that they are normally able to make their own decisions, and every effort must be made to help them. For children, the assumption is that they will increasingly be able to make their own decisions as they grow up, but this is balanced by the responsibilities of parents and the duties of the court to uphold the child's best interests. For both groups, though, it all depends on the specifics of the matter.

Capacity and competence are variable rather than fixed notions, and have to be assessed in the circumstances of each case. All this can make for considerable uncertainty, despite the image that the law brings certainty to uncertain situations.

Questions for reflection

- Look back to questions about the case of MM asked earlier in the chapter (page 89). Having read the rest of the chapter, what do you think now? How far should people be supported (not just allowed) to make choices that may well be harmful to them? Consider the four ethical schools and the four approaches to freedom. What are the implications for you as a social worker?

- Look back to questions about the teenager's choice to refuse treatment, in Box 7.3. Imagine that the case involves a young person you know well. Does that personal connection affect how you think about things? What are the implications for you as a social worker?

Useful websites and further reading

Office of the Public Guardian: www.publicguardian.gov.uk

SCIE Mental Capacity Act Resource: www.scie.org.uk/publications/mca/index.asp

Mental Health Foundation 'assessment of mental capacity audit tool': www.amcat.org.uk

Brown and Barber (2008) *The Social Worker's Guide to the Mental Capacity Act 2005.*

DH (2007) *Independence, Choice and Risk: A Guide to Best Practice in Supported Decision-Making.*

DH (2010a) *Practical Approaches to Safeguarding and Personalisation.*

Mandelstam, M. (2011) *Safeguarding Adults at Risk of Harm: A Legal Guide for Practitioners*, SCIE Report 50, available via the SCIE website.

NIMHE (National Institute for Mental Health in England) (2009) *The Legal Aspects of the Care and Treatment of Children and Young People with Mental Disorder: A Guide for Professionals.*

8 Responsibility and circumstances

> *To what extent should individuals be held responsible for what they do, and how much allowance should be made for mitigating circumstances such as poverty and troubled backgrounds?*

The previous chapter considered questions about the capacity and competence of individuals to make their own decisions, even if these place them in situations of risk. This chapter, and the one that follows, look at another aspect of this difficult weighing up of freedom, risk and protection. This is the issue of responsibility, and how far people should be held responsible for their actions and the outcomes. There are two aspects. This chapter addresses the first of them, namely the balance between holding people responsible and making allowance for difficult circumstances. Chapter 9 considers a related question,

Chapter 9

the relationship between responsibility and blame – specifically, if and when things go wrong, and people suffer harm, how far should the workers who have tried to help them be held to blame?

Chapters
10 & 13

There are close links between these two questions and the chapters should be considered a pair. Both focus on cases of child abuse and neglect, partly because these are matters of such high public profile, but also because they illustrate so well the complexities of untangling different aspects of responsibility. The same issues, though, arise in all other areas of social work – for example, individuals' responsibility for criminal behaviour (discussed in Chapter 10), and workers' responsibilities for ensuring that service users' rights are upheld (Chapter 13).

When we consider the question of parental responsibility for harm suffered by their children, there are three aspects to unravel. There is responsibility in the sense of having caused something, whether or not one is blameworthy for it ('causal responsibility'); responsibility in the sense of being blameworthy ('culpability'); and when or whether responsibility (culpability) should be limited because of mitigating circumstances. Social workers will want to take circumstances into account, but the difficulty of making too many allowances is that this may leave children at risk of harm.

Responsibility and mitigating circumstances

Most of the children and families who receive social work services are likely to be facing very great difficulties in their lives. It is long-established that most will be poor (e.g. Bebbington and Miles, 1989; Parton, 1985, 1991; Stevenson, 2007), as well as facing other challenges such as physical or mental ill-health, learning disabilities, domestic violence, and drug and alcohol problems. The impact of poverty on parenting is shown in Ghate and Hazel's (2002) study of parents living in areas with high levels of material and social disadvantage. The researchers interviewed over 1,750 parents, over the period 1997 to 1999. They found that poor parents were likely to suffer from considerably worse physical and mental health than those who were financially better off. They concluded that the struggle of coping on a low income underlies many of the difficulties that the parents face (see also Katz *et al.*, 2007).

Recent evidence of the extent and depth of the problems facing families involved in care proceedings comes from a study by Masson *et al.* (2008). The study had a sample of 386 cases, involving 682 children, starting care proceedings in the courts in 2004. The researchers comment on the range and multiplicity of problems that the parents were facing. Taking the issues of mental illness, drug and alcohol abuse, learning disabilities, domestic violence and chaotic lifestyle, they found that nearly three-quarters of the mothers had experienced between one and three of them.

There are similar findings in Brandon *et al.*'s studies of serious case reviews in England (2008, 2009, 2010). Serious case reviews are local enquiries into cases where children have died or been seriously injured, and abuse or neglect is known or suspected. Brandon and her colleagues have studied reviews over the periods 2003–5 (161 cases: Brandon *et al.*, 2008), 2005–7 (189 cases: Brandon *et al.*, 2009), and 2007–9 (268 cases: Brandon *et al.*, 2010), giving a total of 618 cases over six years. In summarising their three reports, the researchers highlight a 'toxic trio' of domestic violence, parental mental ill health and parental substance misuse, which often co-exist. These factors are often compounded by poverty, housing problems and parents' own past experiences of ill-treatment, troubled relationships and instability (Brandon *et al.*, 2010: 53–4). In this context, what does it mean to hold parents responsible, and how much allowance should one make for such difficult circumstances?

Of course, some cases are truly ghastly and the harm inflicted on children goes far beyond anything that can be explained by poverty or difficult circumstances – the cases of Victoria Climbié and Baby Peter are striking examples (Laming, 2003; Haringey LSCB, 2009). It is important to remember that most poor people do not ill-treat their children. Difficult circumstances increase the risks, but do not make harm inevitable. Many of the parents make considerable efforts to ensure that their children have the best opportunities possible, and most cases are not like the awful ones that hit the news headlines. In most cases the children stay at home and are kept safe.

It is also worth bearing in mind that even the awful cases are not quite the same as they are presented in the popular press, which simplifies and distorts the complex and difficult realities. Indeed, even the official inquiries tend to simplify and distort the realities of the cases, and the complex requirements of law, policy and practice (Parton, 2004; Sinclair and Corden, 2005; Masson, 2006). This is not to deny that sometimes, with the benefit of hindsight, it is possible to see missed opportunities and predictable mistakes (that is, decisions or practice which has been noted before, in previous inquiries, as contributing to poor outcomes). But the fact that the pitfalls are well known and still happen suggests that they are not as easy to solve as the inquiries sometimes make out.

The popular and political reaction to child abuse tragedies tends to be one of blaming the workers involved (discussed further in the next chapter). There are usually calls for more rules and regulations, and more insistent, authoritative and even authoritarian approaches to the families. The Baby Peter report calls on workers to have a 'healthy scepticism' towards parents (Haringey LSCB, 2009: para. 2.7.5), and the Climbié report uses the term 'respectful uncertainty' (Laming, 2003: para. 6.602). This is not a new issue. The Jasmine Beckford inquiry in 1985, discussed in Box 1.1, also called for social workers to be less trusting of parents and to make greater use of authority (Brent, 1985: 294–5). The studies by Masson *et al.* and Brandon *et al.* described above note frequent lack of parental cooperation with agencies. Brandon *et al.* (2009: 3, 76) list the forms this can take: 'deliberate deception, disguised compliance and "telling workers what they want to hear", selective engagement, and sporadic, passive or desultory compliance'. They conclude that social workers have to be careful in case 'efforts not to be judgemental become a failure to exercise professional judgement' (Brandon *et al.*, 2009: 27).

Certainly social workers have to realise that people may sometimes try to deceive them. But it seems unlikely that suspicion is the best way to build effective relationships with parents that help to keep children safe, and help them to exercise their parental responsibilities more effectively (Sinclair and Corden, 2005). It has to be an attitude that combines compassion with an open and questioning mindset (Brandon *et al.*, 2010: 54; and see Ferguson, 2011). Trying to get the right balance between these two sides is a very demanding practical aspect of the debates about rights and responsibilities discussed in Chapters 1 and 2. How far should parents be *helped* to be responsible and when should they be *held* responsible?

Chapters 1 & 2

Parents' responsibilities, rights and the law

In thinking about parent's responsibilities, their rights, the rights of the children and the duties of the social worker, it is first necessary to distinguish between civil law and criminal law, as discussed in Chapter 3. If there is evidence that parents have committed criminal offences, then they may be charged and sent to criminal trial. In some cases this will clearly be the right thing to do. In others it will be more problematic, if it means that the parents and child will be separated and the child may feel as though he/she is being punished, or if the prosecution fails and the child feels that he/she was not believed (Masson, 2006). Furthermore, social workers are not police officers or prosecutors. They do not investigate crimes or bring criminal proceedings. Child and family social workers make assessments of children in need and their families (DH *et al.*, 2000), and work with other agencies to

Chapter 3

safeguard children (HM Government, 2010c). This may require them to work closely with the police, notably in conducting video-recorded interviews with children (see the detailed guidance in MoJ *et al.*, 2011), but the police have the responsibility for the criminal investigation, not the social worker (HM Government, 2010c: 154–7).

The law requires local authorities to work with families to help them bring up their own children, as far as is consistent with the child's welfare (s. 17 of the Children Act 1989). The first priority is always to try to work in partnership with the parents. This is reinforced by Article 8 of the ECHR, which requires that any interference in private and family life must be in accordance with the law, necessary and proportionate. But Article 8 has to be balanced against Article 3, the unqualified right to be free from inhuman and degrading treatment; and Article 6, the right to a fair hearing. Social workers cannot simply rush in and remove the child from the family. In fact, they have no legal powers to remove a child against the parents' wishes. In an emergency the police can assist by exercising police powers of protection, which last for up to 72 hours. To keep a child in care beyond that, the social worker either has to reach an agreement with the parents or apply to court.

Even when a child is looked after by the local authority (usually in foster care or residential care), the parents retain 'parental responsibility' (PR, loosely defined in s. 3 of the Children Act 1989 as 'all the rights, duties, powers, responsibilities and authority which by law a parent has in relation to the child and his property'). If the child is accommodated under s. 20 of the Act, the local authority does not have PR at all, and arrangements for the child's care have to be made in conjunction with the parent(s) (if they are available). If the child is on a care order (s. 31) the authority shares PR with the parents, although it has the greater weight and is able to overrule the parents on most aspects, but only if necessary (s. 33). However irresponsible the parents may have been, they still retain legal parental responsibility. The expectation on the local authority is that it will still try to work with them. Further, under either legal category, the first priority for the child's placement is to place them back with their parents, and second with other family members (s. 22C; HM Government, 2010b).

The difficulty is that the parents' rights to help in fulfilling their responsibilities can run counter to the child's rights of a timely decision about their future, and a safe and secure upbringing. The problem of delay in child care cases is well known – delay before a case comes to court, during the proceedings, and afterwards, in finding a suitable placement for the child. Delay in care proceedings has been the subject of numerous official reviews and working parties, many recommendations and procedural changes (e.g. Booth, 1996; LCD, 2002, 2003; Brophy, 2006; DfES *et al.*, 2006; Judiciary for England and Wales, 2008; for academic research and critique, see for example Beckett, 2001; McKeigue and Beckett, 2004, 2010; Masson, 2010). For all the endeavour, the duration and cost of care proceedings remain high.

The most recent attempt to address the problems was the Family Justice Review of 2010–11 (chaired by David Norgrove: FJR, 2011a, b). The final report of the Review (November 2011) reported that care cases ending in the first six months of 2011 had taken, on average, 61 weeks in county courts (these would usually be more complex cases) and 48 weeks in the family proceedings courts (magistrates' courts). Like most averages this disguises great variation. Some cases will have taken much longer, even in excess of two years (Cassidy and Davey, 2011), and there is also considerable variation between different parts of the country (FJR, 2011b: 103–4).

There are many reasons for the delays, but prominent amongst them are repeated chances for the parents to make the required changes, and extra assessments (Masson *et al.*, 2008; Cassidy and Davey, 2011). The Family Justice Review identified two major factors behind them: a culture of mistrust between local authorities and the courts, and an awareness, from all sides, of the extreme seriousness of the decisions to be made. Together, these lead to routine commissioning of new assessments, duplication of work and 'a vicious cycle of inefficiency and delay' (FJR, 2011a: 101).

To tackle the problem, the Review called for a more proportionate degree of scrutiny from the courts. This would mean that they cut back on overly detailed scrutiny of the care plan, to focus instead on the essentials, and stop ordering further assessments as a matter of course. It proposed a statutory time limit of six months for care proceedings, save for exceptions – the difficulty, of course, is to decide what counts as an exception. The final report offered guidelines on this, which allow for testing a placement back with parents or family, a significant and unforeseeable change of circumstances, and unusual complexity (FJR, 2011b: 108). The trouble is that these are precisely the sorts of issues that already contribute to delay, and it is hard to see how this list will effectively restrict the number of exceptions.

The Family Justice Review final report commented that most respondents to their consultation supported the call for a six month time limit, and the government accepted it (MoJ and DfE, 2012). There are certainly many opposed to it, and warnings that it could lead to miscarriages of justice if the evidence is not tested thoroughly or options explored fully (see Pemberton, 2012a). Whether and how it will be achieved remains to be seen. The following comment from the Review summarises the problem, but in doing so shows why change will be hard to achieve:

> Understandable sympathy for parents and an acute awareness of the enormity of the decisions encourages a wish to explore every avenue. The idea of a proportionate approach comes across

as unfeeling as well as seeming to risk denial of the parents' right to a fair hearing. Processes become exhaustive so that when a decision is finally made everyone can be reassured that everything that could be done was done. We were told and we agree that the right of the parents to a fair hearing has come too often to override the paramount welfare of the child.

(FJR, 2011b: 92)

Care proceedings

The courts regard care orders as an extreme measure and even though the civil law test is the balance of probabilities, they still require strong evidence and clear plans. The criteria for a care order are demanding, and are shown in Boxes 8.1 and 8.2. The courts certainly do not see themselves merely as a rubber stamp for the local authorities, but take their duties of scrutinising the case very seriously. (This can be seen from two judgments about applications for emergency protection orders, discussed later in the chapter.)

Box 8.1: Care proceedings: eight requirements

Before a court can make a care order, it has to be satisfied on eight matters. The first of these are known as the 'threshold criteria', in s. 31 of the Children Act 1989. If these are not met, the court cannot make the order. Even if they are, it does not have to make a care order. That will depend on how it assesses the other matters.

1   **The threshold criteria:**

    s. 31(2) A court may only make a care order or a supervision order if it is satisfied:

    (a) that the child is suffering or likely to suffer significant harm; and

    (b) that the harm, or likelihood of harm, is attributable to:

        (i)   the care given to the child, or likely to be given to him, not being what it would be reasonable to expect a parent to give him; or

        (ii) the child's being beyond parental control.

Plus the 'welfare tests' in s. 1 of the Children Act 1989:

2   **Welfare principle** – the child's welfare is the court's 'paramount consideration' (but note, not the only consideration).

3   **Minimum delay principle** (but 'planned and purposeful' delay is allowed).

---

4   **No order principle** (the court shall not make an order unless it considers doing so would be better for the child than not. The implication is that there must be a clear and convincing plan for the child).

5   **The items on the welfare checklist** (see Box 8.2).

And:

6   **Human Rights Act 1998 and ECHR rights** – that the order is legally justified, necessary and proportionate (Articles 3, 6 and 8 are especially relevant).

7   **Contact arrangements for children on care orders** – s. 34(11).

8   **The care plan** – s. 31A.

Box 8.2: Care proceedings: the welfare checklist

Section 1(3) of the Children Act 1989 contains a list of factors to which the court must have particular regard when deciding whether to make a care or supervision order. The items on the list have considerable implications for social work policy, planning and practice.

*   *The ascertainable wishes and feelings of the child, considered in the light of their age and understanding* (the implication for social workers is to get to know the child, to find these out and to understand them).

*   *The physical, emotional and educational needs of the child* (the implication is to be clear what these are, and have a plan how to meet them).

*   *The likely effect of any change* (the implication is to have a plan how to help the child deal with any potentially difficult consequences, such as being separated from their siblings or carers).

*   *Age, sex, background and other characteristics of the child* (these might include the child's ethnicity, culture and language – and as always, the point is to be clear about what these mean for the child, for their day-to-day experience of life, and how any needs arising from them will be met).

*   *Any harm suffered/at risk of suffering* (the implication is to have a plan to reduce any harmful effects, or to reduce the risk).

- *The capabilities of the parent(s) and relevant others* (the implication is to have assessed these carefully, including non-resident parents and members of the extended family, and to have offered suitable support).

- *The range of powers available to the court* (the implication is that social workers will need to consider all those options too, and be able to explain why they are not as suitable as the plan they are proposing).

There has been a substantial and sustained increase in the number of care applications since the Baby Peter case in November 2008. The number of applications rose from 6,488 in 2008–9 to 10,225 in 2011–12 (see the 'care statistics' page on the Cafcass website. Note that this is the number of cases, rather than the number of children. Cafcass is the Child and Family Courts Advisory and Support Service, the body that employs children's guardians. These are social workers who are appointed in care proceedings to review the local authority's plans and make an independent report to the court about the child's welfare). It is important to appreciate that local authorities still deal with the majority of cases outside care proceedings, even when the children are considered to be at risk of significant harm. In these cases, it is likely that the children will be on child protection plans, and on 31 March 2011 there were 42,700 children on such plans in England (DfE, 2011b). These children will have been discussed at an inter-agency child protection case conference, which will have decided that there was a likelihood of significant harm, but other factors (say, a degree of parental cooperation) meant that an application to court was not necessary, and an inter-agency plan was sufficient (HM Government, 2010c: 167–70).

So, social workers will often be working with children who are suffering or likely to suffer significant harm, often because of neglect (42 per cent of those on child protection plans are because of neglect, the largest category: DfE, 2011b). Many will be living in impoverished and deprived circumstances, and social workers may be involved with the families over long periods of time, often years (perhaps 'on and off', with the case being closed and then re-opened, or changes of worker). Often these cases 'bump along the bottom', which creates a difficulty for taking them to court. Given that social workers have known the family for so long, and considered it acceptable to leave the child at home, what has changed now that justifies going to court? This can be a hard issue to prove unless there has been a sudden change or a dramatic incident, so the tendency is to wait for such an event, a 'catapult' (Dickens, 2007; and see Iwaniec *et al.*, 2004; Buckley, 2005; Stevenson, 2007). One reason that has been suggested for the recent increase in care proceedings is that social workers are now more aware of the harms of neglect, and so are more ready to start court action (Pemberton, 2012b). Even so, it is likely that the case will have been known to children's services for a long time. Then, when the case does get to court, the local authority is likely to be criticised for leaving it so long, which feeds into the culture of mistrust described above.

Neglect cases also take us back to the question of responsibility and mitigating circumstances. They raise this especially sharply because of the close links with poverty, making it hard to say what is attributable to individual choices and behaviour, and what is attributable to deprived circumstances. It has been described as a 'chicken and egg' relationship, where it is impossible to say which comes first (McSherry, 2004; see also McSherry, 2007).

Whatever the causes, it is important for social workers to be clear and realistic about the possibilities and the timescales for change. Ward *et al*'s (2010) study of children who were identified as having suffered or being at risk of suffering significant harm before their first birthdays found that professionals tried everything they could to keep families together, often giving the parents repeated opportunities to show that they could look after the child. Yet Ward *et al*'s salutary finding is that unless parental change happens very quickly, it is unlikely to happen. In their study, all but one of the parents who made sufficient changes did so before the baby was six months old. They warn against over-optimistic assessments, particularly from experts such as psychologists, psychiatrists and independent social workers. Two-thirds of these recommended that the child stay with the parents, but in over half of these cases the children eventually had to be removed. Similarly, Farmer and Lutman (2010), in a study of neglected children returned to their birth families, found over-optimistic views of parental capacity to change, especially from experts and children's guardians in court proceedings. They also emphasise the importance of realistic assessment and planning, and proactive case management and review.

Emergency protection

A court may make an emergency protection order (EPO) on the application of any person (not just a local authority), if is satisfied that there is reasonable cause to believe that the child concerned is likely to suffer significant harm unless they are removed to a safe place, or kept in a safe place (for example, a hospital or a foster home) (Children Act 1989, s. 44). It allows the applicant to place or keep the child away from their parents for up to eight days, if this is necessary for his/her welfare. It also gives the applicant parental responsibility for the child, but they may only exercise this to the extent that is reasonable given the short-term nature of the order.

The conditions for getting an EPO are much lower than for a care order – the court only has to be satisfied that there is 'reasonable cause to believe' the conditions are met. It does not have to decide about the causes of the risk, whether it is attributable to shortcomings in parental care – the simple fact of the likelihood is enough, and the welfare checklist does not apply. Compared to a care order, then, it is a much reduced test. This does not mean, however, that the courts regard making an EPO as a minor matter. This can be seen from the judgment in the case of *X Council v B (Emergency Protection Orders)* [2004], shown in Box 8.3.

Box 8.3: Emergency protection orders: guiding principles

In the case of *X Council v B (Emergency Protection Orders)* [2004], Mr Justice Munby strongly criticised the way that a local authority had applied for and implemented an EPO. In paragraph 57 of his judgment he summarised the key principles that should apply (subsequently endorsed in the case of *Re X (Emergency Protection Orders)* [2006]). The main points, using Mr Justice Munby's words, are:

- An EPO, summarily removing a child from his parents, is a 'draconian' and 'extremely harsh' measure, requiring 'exceptional justification' and 'extraordinarily compelling reasons'. Such an order should not be made unless the court is satisfied that it is both necessary and proportionate and that no other less radical form of order will achieve the essential end of promoting the welfare of the child. Separation is only to be contemplated if immediate separation is essential to secure the child's safety; 'imminent danger' must be 'actually established'.

- It is important that both the local authority and the court approach every application for an EPO with an anxious awareness of the extreme gravity of the relief being sought and a scrupulous regard for the Convention rights of both the child and the parents.

- Any order must provide for the least interventionist solution consistent with the preservation of the child's immediate safety.

- No EPO should be made for any longer than is absolutely necessary to protect the child.

- The evidence in support of the application for an EPO must be full, detailed, precise and compelling.

- Save in wholly exceptional cases, parents must be given adequate prior notice of the date, time and place of any application by a local authority for an EPO.

- The local authority must apply its mind very carefully to whether removal is essential in order to secure the child's immediate safety. The mere fact that the local authority has obtained an EPO is not of itself enough . . . The local authority, even after it has obtained an EPO, is under an obligation to consider less drastic alternatives to emergency removal.

- . . . sections 44(10)(a) and 44(11)(a) [of the Children Act 1989] impose on the local authority a mandatory obligation to return a child who it has removed . . . if 'it appears to [the local authority] that it is safe for the child to be returned'. This imposes on the local authority a continuing duty to keep the case under review day by day . . . In this, as in other respects, the local authority is under a duty to exercise exceptional diligence.

- Section 44(13) requires the local authority, subject only to any direction given by the court, to allow a child who is subject to an EPO 'reasonable contact' with his parents. Arrangements for contact must be driven by the needs of the family, not stunted by lack of resources.

A further example of the thorough scrutiny that the courts give to local authority actions and plans is the case of a baby boy known in the court proceedings as 'K'. His mother was referred to as 'G' and his father as 'C'. This was another case heard by Mr Justice Munby. There were a number of hearings: 30 January 2008 (*R (G) v Nottingham City Council* [2008]); 18 February 2008 (*R (G) v Nottingham City Council No. 2* [2008]); and 14 March 2008 (*Re K (Child), Nottingham City Council v G and others* [2008]). There is also a report into the case by Nottingham City Safeguarding Children Board (2009), and a judgment given in criminal proceedings against the mother in 2009 (reported in *This is Nottingham*, 2009). G was identified by name in the criminal case.

In early 2008, G was 18 years old and expecting a baby at the beginning of February. She had had an unhappy and troubled childhood, and had been in care to Nottingham City Council. This meant they had a duty to continue supporting her, and to prepare a 'pathway plan' as to how they would do so. G's lawyers considered the assessment and the plan so inadequate that they had applied for judicial review. This was due to be heard at the High Court in London on 30 January 2008. The day before, G went into labour. She gave birth at about 2am on 30 January, and a few hours later her baby was removed from her by the midwife, in accordance with a birth plan made in December 2007. When the judicial review hearing opened, her lawyer applied for an order to reunite them, arguing that the separation was unlawful because it was without G's agreement or any legal authorisation. There was no EPO or interim care order, the child was not under police protection, and there was no medical need or urgent crisis to justify immediate separation (if there were, this could have been done under s. 3(5) of the Children Act 1989). The local authority accepted this, and the judge made an order that G and K be reunited provided they stayed in the hospital. They were reunited shortly afterwards. The same day, the local authority applied to court in Nottingham for an interim care order on K, which was granted. K was then lawfully removed from G and placed in a foster home. The criticism was not that Nottingham had acted without good cause, but that they acted unlawfully.

More details of what had happened came out in the later hearings and the Nottingham City review. According to the local authority, G knew about the plan in advance and did not oppose it, and did not object when the midwife told her that the separation was about to happen (G said that she had frequently raised objections). It was accepted that G had not given actual consent to the separation, but the local authority had treated the absence of objection as sufficient. Mr Justice Munby was highly critical of this, because G had given birth such a short time before she was required to make this decision. There was also the context of G's troubled circumstances and history of not working well with social services (see the second judgment, paras 42–64). The judge commented that 'Submission in the face of asserted state authority is not the same as consent. In this context . . . nothing short of consent will suffice' (para. 61). He held that the separation had been unlawful under English law and in breach of Article 8 of the ECHR.

Meanwhile, the care proceedings continued. They had been transferred to the High Court and reserved to Mr Justice Munby. With the agreement of the local authority he gave a direction under s. 38(6) of the Children Act that there should be a residential assessment of G and K at a specialist mother and baby unit, possibly to be joined later by K's father, C. G went there by herself for a fortnight's initial assessment. At the end of the first week she went home as planned, but after that refused to return.

G and C had been having contact with K, although the quality of the visits was described as very poor, with them putting their own needs ahead of K's. On 12 March there was a contact visit when G and C had a violent argument, fighting physically with K in between them. The contact supervisor asked G to give K to her, and G threw him at her from a distance of about 18 inches (described in the judgment of the hearing held on 14 March 2008, para. 16). This was in the middle of a fight, K was only six weeks old and his head was not supported. In these circumstances the residential assessment was abandoned, and the local authority given a time-limited order allowing them to refuse contact between G and K.

Later, in February 2009, G was convicted of child cruelty and sentenced to a two-year community order with supervision. By then, K was due to be placed for adoption and G was pregnant again, but not expecting to keep the baby. The judge in the criminal trial noted that G was damaged and vulnerable as a result of her upbringing, but still held her responsible for her own conduct. He said:

> It is well documented that the social services department acted unlawfully in removing your child from you. All they did that was inappropriate was that they took the child from you before they obtained a court order. Your subsequent conduct clearly demonstrates beyond any doubt at all that the instinct and judgment of the social workers was entirely correct.
>
> (His Honour Judge Stokes, quoted in *This is Nottingham*, 2009)

Conclusion

The chapter has considered the challenges of protecting children whilst taking account of parents' circumstances and rights. How can parents be helped to exercise their responsibilities, and when must they be held responsible? These are two sides of the same coin. Social workers are charged with safeguarding children, and supporting parents. To do that they have to try to work with the parents in context, which means understanding their needs and rights, but not being diverted into losing focus on the child. Similarly, the courts are charged with promoting the welfare of children and ensuring that parents' responsibilities and rights are upheld. Even when there are strong grounds for concern, due legal process must be followed, and that takes account of the rights of the parents as well as the welfare of children.

Trying to do all things at the same time will inevitably lead, from time to time, to disagreements between the various professionals and agencies involved. This is not necessarily because any of them are acting unreasonably or in anything less than good faith, but because they all have their own professional duties *and* their own competing responsibilities to meet, to safeguard children and to support parents (Dickens, 2004, 2005). It is the old debate from the1980s (Box 1.1.), as live today as it ever was.

At the present time, the tensions seem especially tight. There are loud demands to be more sceptical of parents, to limit the number of chances given to them, to conclude care cases more swiftly, to move children through to adoption more speedily. At the same time, there are also calls to develop more preventive services, and more community-based and empowering ways of working with families. This is not just the call of radicals and academics (e.g. Ferguson and Woodward, 2009; Ayre and Preston-Shoot, 2010; Mantle and Backwith, 2011; Lavalette, 2011), but also a professed priority for the current coalition government (e.g. Field, 2010; Allen, 2011; Munro, 2011b; DfE, 2011a). At the same time as all this talk, cuts in government funding to local authorities and other agencies (such as Sure Start children's centres: Watt, 2011), are making it very hard to sustain such services.

In summary, it is not nearly as straightforward as newspaper columnists, politicians and even some social work commentators sometimes say to 'rescue' children from harmful situations. This is an issue that we take further in the following chapter.

Questions for reflection

- Look back to the definition of parental responsibility on page 101. What sort of things would you include in it? You may find it interesting to compare your answer with a list given in a government guide for parents who are separating, *Parenting Plans: Putting Your Children First* (DCSF and Cafcass, 2008: 35).

- Think about a family you have worked with. How well were the parents fulfilling their responsibilities? What was making it hard for them? What help were they getting?

- Does the law offer too many safeguards to parents? What, if anything, would you change?

Useful websites and further reading

SCIE e-learning site on poverty, parenting and social exclusion: www.scie.org.uk/publications/elearning/poverty/index.asp

Cafcass (Children and Family Courts Advisory and Support Service): www.cafcass.gov.uk/

Katz *et al.* (2007) *The Relationship Between Parenting and Poverty.*

Stevenson (2007) *Neglected Children and their Families.*

Ferguson (2011) *Child Protection Practice.*

Davies and Ward (2011) *Safeguarding Children Across Services: Messages from Research*, available via the DfE website: www.education.gov.uk/publications/eOrderingDownload/DFE-RR164.pdf.

9 Responsibility and blame

Imagine you are the social worker for a child who is the subject of a child protection plan. There have been a number of inter-agency child protection case conferences. There is known to be a risk to the child, but the decision – based on your assessment, and which you supported – was that the child should remain at home. The child is killed. Are you responsible?

The question of social workers' responsibility for sad outcomes raises hard questions about the different dimensions of responsibility – personal, professional, organisational and legal. It also raises questions about the nature of social work's expertise – how certain can we ever be about our decisions? – and about the multi-agency, inter-professional aspects of the job. These are perennial challenges for social work, coming up especially painfully whenever a child abuse scandal hits the news headlines, but always there in the background. They take us to the heart of debates about the balance between social workers' individual responsibility, organisational factors, and the wider political and social context.

Before reading further, take some time to think about the answer – or perhaps better, answers – to the question above, about the social worker's responsibility. A number of sub-questions arise: is the social worker blameworthy? Is the 'rightness' of a decision or action dependent on the outcome? Are there different sorts of responsibility?

Is the social worker blameworthy?

There may be questions here about how well the social worker did their assessment. Did they speak to all the right people, gather all the necessary information, and evaluate it accurately? If there are shortcomings the social worker may well find themselves being held responsible, but is that really fair? Such questions were carefully explored in a series of articles linked with the child abuse scandals of the 1980s (see Box 1.1). The start was a provocative paper by Hollis and Howe (1987) on moral risks in social work. They concluded that the social worker is morally responsible for cases that turn out badly: 'The failures are not hers alone but hers they remain … That is to give her all the greater credit for moral courage … children can be grateful for brave people, who are willing to take the moral risk' (Hollis and Howe, 1987: 134). The article provoked a reply by Macdonald (1990a), a response by Hollis and Howe (1990) and a final reply by Macdonald (1990b). Although the first of those papers is over 25 years old now, the debates are as pertinent as ever. There are a number of points to be made.

Shared responsibility

First, to pick up the point that 'the failures are not hers alone'. Social workers very rarely make decisions by themselves. Assessments are likely to involve other professionals as well as social workers, and social workers' reports and recommendations are likely to be reviewed by their own managers and other professionals. Rather than see it as an individual responsibility, perhaps it is better treated as a shared one. Even so, a responsibility shared is not a responsibility shed (Hollis and Howe, 1987: 132), and it is important that social workers (like any employee) do not try to deny their part.

It is often assumed that inter-professional and inter-agency working will produce fuller information and better assessments, but experience shows that is not necessarily so. Mistakes and misjudgments by one professional can mislead others. In the case of Victoria Climbié, for example, a doctor diagnosed the marks on her body as scabies, not signs of non-accidental injury (Laming, 2003). In the case of Baby Peter, he had been on a child protection plan for over eighteen months at the time of his death, involving inter-agency working. He had been seen by numerous health professionals as well as social care staff (this included hospital staff, his family doctor, health visitor and consultant paediatrician: Haringey LSCB, 2009).

In the scenario at the start of the chapter, the decision to leave the child at home was made in a multi-disciplinary meeting. Again, the assumption is that such meetings pool information and lead to better decisions, but that may not always happen. In Peter's case, the report of the second serious case review comments that the majority of attendees at his initial case conference were not specialists in child safeguarding work, and there was tendency to minimise the significance of the injuries (Haringey LSCB, 2009: para. 3.8.5). (Note: the report of the first serious case review was rejected for not being sufficiently rigorous, but both have since been published on the Department for Education website: Haringey LSCB, 2008 and 2009). The local authority has the primary legal and professional responsibility for child safeguarding, and the report maintains that the chairperson should have provided clearer guidance to the non-specialists. Further, the presence of Peter's mother and her solicitor at the conference may have inhibited the discussion. The chair could have asked for them to withdraw for a period of time (Haringey LSCB, 2009: para 3.8.26).

Bureaucracy

Second, there are so many regulations and procedures to follow in cases like this, so many rules about what should be done and when, that in the busy-ness of highly pressured, under-resourced social work teams, it is almost inevitable that something will have been missed out (Macdonald, 1990a; Howe, 1992). Indeed, taking some short cuts (intentionally or unintentionally) is often the only way that the work can get done at all (Sinclair and Corden, 2005). Under the day-to-day pressures of the work, following the rule book to the letter is likely to lead to criticism of inflexibility, slowness and defensive practice; but after the event, the short cuts are held up as shortcomings.

A major review of the child protection system in England was commissioned by the coalition government shortly after the general election of 2010. It was led by Professor Eileen Munro, and produced three reports in 2010–11 (Munro, 2010, 2011a, 2011b). One of the strongly made points was that the proliferation of procedures has created a highly bureaucratic system that actually makes it harder to keep a focus on the well-being of the children. Moreover, it has undermined social workers' sense of professional responsibility (e.g. Munro, 2011b: 137). This has in turn reduced job satisfaction and contributed to high sickness rates and high staff turnover, thus making it harder for those who are left to focus on the needs of the children – a vicious cycle.

Munro's challenge is to reclaim professional responsibility, and to build a new culture in children's services, a learning culture rather than a compliance culture. This would allow professional judgment to be exercised effectively, with (most importantly) proper guidance and support for social workers to do so (Munro, 2011b: 7). Her call is for clearer roles rather than more rules. This will certainly be a big change for social work in England, where public outrage against social workers is so great when there is a child abuse death, and where the standard response for so long has been to add more rules and procedures. It is hard to envisage how such a juggernaut can be turned round, not least because many social workers as well as their critics like the apparent security of the rules, rather than the risks of professional judgment (even though, in reality, any security they offer frequently proves to be an illusion).

Moral luck

Third is the fact that misfortune happens. In the scenario, as in real life, there are known to be risks in leaving the child at home. That is why the child is on a child protection plan. But in any situation where there are risks, sooner or later the risk will occur. Even if the odds against the event happening are a million to one, someone, sooner or later, will have the millionth case. They need not have done anything wrong, they may have assessed everything properly and followed every rule – they just got the unlucky case.

A possible response is to say that this is not quite a matter of random luck. After all, there is known to be a risk. That implies that with more care, it could have been identified and prevented. But that in turn leads us on to the limitations of social work expertise and assessment tools. Certainly there are factors which are known to increase the risks for children, most notably parental drug misuse, domestic violence and mental ill-health, but there are no guaranteed predictors of serious injury or death, or any guaranteed combination (Brandon *et al.*, 2010: 53). Social work is not an exact science, but deals with messy situations and unpredictable human lives. However many procedures, however detailed the guidelines, there will always be some cases that are missed. Rules and frameworks, like ethical codes, try to bring certainty, but complete certainty is an illusory goal. Social workers are left to deal with uncertainty

On that point, it is worth noting that the scenario does not say how the child died. It may be that she was killed by her parents, but it could have been an accident, an illness or a long-standing health condition. Children on child protection plans sometimes die from such causes. It is likely that the circumstances of the child's death will be carefully investigated. It is possible that the child was not properly supervised or cared for, but also it is possible that there will be no cause to hold the parents or the social worker responsible.

Without doubt all workers and managers involved in cases where children (or adults) die or are seriously harmed, feel great regret and sadness at what happened. But there is a difference between an emotional reaction and a reasoned analysis. An example that shows this is how a driver might feel if a child ran out in front of their car, suddenly and unexpectedly, and they simply could not stop in time. No doubt the driver would feel terrible, but if they were driving legally, paying due attention and so on, that is not the same as being culpable.

But what happens if the brakes were faulty? This is an example debated by Hollis and Howe and Macdonald in their series of papers, and by Banks (2012: 31–2). If the driver had neglected to do proper checks, or drives the car knowing it to be faulty, perhaps they do become culpable. How one answers that, though, may depend on why they chose to drive the car. Hollis and Howe (1990: 550) imagine an ambulance driver being called to an accident. There is only one ambulance, with faulty brakes. The driver has to try to help the injured people, but crashes on the way back and kills them. Is the driver to blame? Hollis and Howe's answer is yes, but in context. It is not the driver's fault alone, but it is still their fault. Macdonald (1990b: 554) disagrees. If the decision was a reasonable one at the time, weighing up the risks and potential benefits, then it was the right decision, even if it had a bad outcome.

How much does outcome matter?

The question here is whether the 'rightness' of a decision or action depends on the outcome. This takes us back to the differences between Kantianism and utilitarianism, a categorical approach and a consequentialist approach. From a Kantian perspective, if something is the right thing to do, it's the right thing to do, regardless of the consequences. So, in the scenario, one would reach a decision about what to do based on the assessment of the case, understanding of the law and the guiding principles of ethical action. Kant expresses these principles in terms of treating everyone involved as an end not only as a means, and asking whether one could, logically, wish it to be a universal rule that similar cases are dealt with in the same way. We might translate these into more modern, legal and social work vocabulary, such as respecting the rights of everyone involved, treating people fairly, taking all relevant matters into account and being consistent. At heart these are Kantian values. If, after all that, the child dies, it does not affect the correctness of the decision. If the decision was made in the right way for the right reasons, it remains the right decision, and the person who made it ought not to be blamed.

The consequentialists take a different position, and the rightness of the decision is affected by the outcome. At one level, the death of the child shows it was the wrong decision, as simple as that, and the people involved have to accept their responsibility. But at another level there is a wider view of the consequences. A society in which children are removed from their families whenever there is a problem or a hint of risk, is unlikely to be a happy one in which to live. But taking a risk and leaving children at home means that, sooner or later, some of them will be seriously injured or killed. Sad as that is, it brings more happiness in the long run, because there are important social values about freedom and privacy that should not be overruled except in the most extreme cases. In this sense, the happiness, even the lives, of some children are traded off against happiness of the majority.

The point is that our child welfare system allows more risk – indeed, requires more risk – than it would tolerate if children's safety alone were the sole consideration. It isn't. There are the libertarian values about freedom from state intervention, and relativist values about freedom to follow different lifestyles, as well as the Kantian and utilitarian arguments. And as we saw in the previous chapter, there are also radical arguments against a narrow child-rescue approach – society should be offering more help, sooner, to the most vulnerable families, supporting them not punishing them.

In this sense, then, bad outcomes for some individual children are inevitable. Most inquiries into child abuse deaths make the observation that it is impossible to prevent all deaths or ill-treatment, but then go on to identify the 'mistakes' made on their particular case, which mean (in their view) that this one *could* have been prevented. But it is important to see individual cases in the bigger, social and political context. This was analysed brilliantly by Dingwall *et al.* (1983, 2nd edition 1995), in their study of child protection practice in the late 1970s. Law, policy and organisational structures have changed greatly since then, and there is now much more knowledge about child abuse and neglect, but as Dingwall *et al.* say in the postscript to the second edition, 'the practical problems and moral dilemmas' have remained the same (Dingwall *et al.*, 1995: 245).

Dingwall *et al.* found that there is an 'institutionalised preference for an optimistic version of the events' (1983: 73), and for the least overtly coercive form of intervention. This has three main aspects. First, there is the organisational context, of high workloads and limited resources, which creates a tendency for staff to minimise risk factors and screen out cases that might, if investigated more vigorously, turn out to be ill-treatment. There simply isn't the time to scrutinise everything, so short cuts have to be taken, and explanations accepted at face value until that becomes untenable. Second is the 'division of regulatory labour', the number of different agencies and different professionals involved, with different expertise, experience, status and roles. The list includes social workers and their managers, doctors, teachers, police officers, health visitors and lawyers. The range of different perspectives creates another bias against compulsory intervention. Dingwall *et al.* (1983: 77) describe it as rather like getting three lemons on a gambling machine.

Finally, there is what Dingwall *et al.* call 'the rule of optimism'. This is the idea that the most favourable light will be shed on events and explanations, until that becomes no longer feasible. It has two components – 'natural love' and 'cultural relativism'. The first holds that caring parent–child relationships are a natural fact, so any accusation that this is not the case in a particular family is especially grave, and has to be backed up by strong evidence. The second holds that different styles of child rearing are valid in their own cultural context, and should not be illiberally suppressed unless there is clear evidence that they are harming the child.

The rule of optimism has proved a controversial concept. It has been used to criticise social workers for being naive and unquestioning of parents (as in Brent, 1985), but it is important to appreciate its original meaning. It was not about individual social workers' gullibility, but part of a wider, social and political understanding of child protection work. Given that our society places such high value on freedom and family privacy, state intervention is only allowed on the basis of a compromise that minimises the likelihood of compulsory action.

Different aspects of responsibility

Responsibility in social work has many faces. There are questions of causality, culpability and allowance for circumstances, as much for social workers as for parents (as discussed in Chapter 8). In addition there are legal, organisational, professional and personal dimensions, and there is also the challenge that responsibilities are owed to many different individuals and groups.

Four types of responsibility

This section considers the inter-relationships between four types of responsibility – legal, organisational, professional and personal. These may reinforce one another, or be in conflict, or one aspect might offer some defence against criticism on another.

It may well be that the social worker is not legally responsible; and as we shall see, the law may offer some possibilities for social workers to defend themselves from undue blame. Certainly, the social worker did not kill the child, and is not guilty in that sense. Furthermore, it is the local authority, the organisation, not the individual worker, that carries the legal duty under the Children Act 1989 to safeguard children from harm. The authority also has statutory duties to promote the upbringing of children by their families and to return children to their parents, if appropriate. Deciding how to balance and exercise these duties, especially in the context of high demand and limited resources, involves difficult decisions.

Beyond the statutory duties, social workers and the council have a common law duty of care to the child in child protection investigations (see Chapter 2). If they have been negligent in their handling of the case, there may be grounds for legal action (the action will normally be against the employer, who is vicariously liable for the conduct of their employees). As discussed in Chapter 2, however, the grounds for a finding of negligence are narrow. A claim will not succeed if the social worker's actions are within what is reasonable to expect of a reasonably competent practitioner.

Social workers have another layer of responsibility in terms of their professional duties. They may be answerable to a professional association or a professional regulator. In the UK, BASW is the professional association for social work, but membership is voluntary and most social workers do not belong. In England, a new government-backed College of Social Work came into being at the start of 2012, to promote the profession and raise standards, but it is not the professional regulator. At the time of writing that was the GSCC, and all social workers had to be registered with it and comply with its code of practice, but it was replaced by the Health and Care Professions Council in 2012 (Dickens, 2012).

As for personal responsibility, we noted earlier that feeling regret does not automatically imply blameworthiness. But should workers accept personal responsibility? Decisions are usually shared, as we noted earlier, and many will be shaped by organisational pressures, budgets and workloads, as much as the service user's needs. For all that, it is important to retain a sense of personal responsibility, for social workers to see themselves as moral agents, not just bureaucratic functionaries. It is not good enough to deny responsibility, to say 'I was just following orders' or 'it was all the other person's fault'. Greater evils lie this way, if workers do not resist the erosion of moral responsibility by organisational pressures (Rhodes, 1986; Preston-Shoot, 2010, 2011).

The four ethical approaches all provide steps forward, but none, of course, gives easy answers. Social workers need a strong sense of personal responsibility and duty, and a strong sense of responsibility for the consequences of their actions. They need to retain a sense of care for the people with whom they work, however troubled those people are and even when exercising control. In terms of virtue ethics, the good character finds the middle way between the extremes of denying responsibility and taking unjustified blame. They have a sense of appropriate responsibility, not trying to wriggle off the hook but not prepared to be scapegoated either.

Widely owed responsibilities

There is also the question of who the responsibilities are owed to. Here again there are many aspects, with obligations to the children, parents, colleagues, the employer, the professional regulator, and society more generally. There might well be different obligations to different service users, most notably protecting children and supporting parents; or duties to individuals that sit uneasily with wider duties to society as a whole. Because social workers have so many different types of responsibility, and owe rather imprecise responsibilities to so many different people, it is inevitable that succeeding in some will mean they fail in others.

It is a gloomy conclusion, that social work is a profession with failure guaranteed, but it is not the whole picture. Many children, families and individuals are helped. As we have noted, however, for a whole variety of organisational, professional and societal reasons, not all children can be saved. It takes us back to Hollis and Howe's (1987) argument that social workers should be commended for taking on the risk, not vilified.

The Baby Peter case

For all that, we know that when social workers and their managers are seen to have failed in some aspects of their work, particularly in child protection cases, there is a likelihood that they will be criticised very damningly and very publicly. Some have suffered vicious personal criticism in the media and death threats from members of the public. Some have lost their jobs. In the Baby Peter case, five members of staff were sacked from the children's services department that was responsible for Peter's case, the London Borough of Haringey – the director, two senior managers, the team manager and the social worker.

Peter Connelly died as a result of appalling injuries in August 2007, aged 17 months. The criminal trial of his mother, her boyfriend and his brother ended on 11 November 2008. It had received extensive media coverage, and there was an aggressive campaign by the *Sun* newspaper against the workers involved, demanding that they be sacked. The day after the trial, the Secretary of State for Children, Schools and Families, Ed Balls, ordered a swift review of child safeguarding arrangements in Haringey. This was to be a 'joint area review', to be led by Ofsted (the Office for Standards in Education, the body responsible for inspecting local authority children's services). These normally took five months, but Mr Balls required the report by 1 December, giving less than three weeks. Ofsted produced its final draft report on 30 November. This was highly critical of the systems in Haringey, but (in keeping with their policy and practice) did not criticise any individuals by name. On 1 December, Ed Balls issued a direction to Haringey to remove the director, Sharon Shoesmith, from her post, announcing this in a press conference without any warning to her. The borough subsequently sacked her.

Ms Shoesmith later used the law and the courts to argue that she had been unfairly dismissed. She applied for judicial review, arguing that the way she had been removed from her post and then sacked was unlawful because she was not given a proper chance to put her side of the story (see Chapter 3, on the principles of lawful decision-making). At the first hearing, Ms Shoesmith's application was

dismissed, but she appealed against this and in May 2011 the Court of Appeal decided in her favour, against the Department for Education and Haringey Council (*R (Shoesmith) v Ofsted and others* [2011]). They wanted to appeal against the decision, but in August 2011 the Supreme Court refused them leave to do so.

Ms Shoesmith had been the director, and so there was a chain of organisational accountability up to her. But that did not mean she could be summarily dismissed. As the judge put it, '"Accountability" is not synonymous with "heads must roll"' (para. 66 of the judgment). Being accountable meant that she was entitled to an opportunity to give her account, to a fair hearing. Whether her account would have proved satisfactory is another matter, but judicial reviews focus on the fairness of the decision-making process, not the decision itself. The point is she was not given the chance.

Ms Shoesmith was not a social worker (she came from a teaching background), so she was not answerable to the professional regulator, the GSCC. The social worker, Maria Ward, and her team manager, Gillie Christou, were, so they were accountable both to their employer and to the GSCC. In terms of the former, they were sacked by Haringey for gross misconduct in April 2009. They went to an employment tribunal on the grounds of unfair dismissal in May 2009. The decision was given in October 2010 to reject their case, but in June 2011 they were given permission to appeal against this. The Employment Appeal Tribunal heard the case in February 2012, and announced its decision on 25 May 2012. It rejected their appeal, upholding the decision of the original tribunal. Lawyers for Ms Ward and Ms Christou said that they were considering whether to try to take the matter further, to the Court of Appeal. That had not been decided at the time of writing, so watch out for further developments in this case.

In terms of professional accountability, they were both suspended from the GSCC register on an interim basis in December 2008. Their cases were heard together by the GSCC conduct committee in May 2010. The official notifications of the decisions are publicly available on the GSCC website (GSCC, 2010a, 2010b). Both of them admitted misconduct, and were held to be in breach of various elements in the GSCC code of practice for social care workers.

Neither was struck off the register permanently. Ms Ward was suspended for 18 months in total, which meant she had two months more to serve. Ms Christou, as the manager, was suspended for 20 months, which meant she had four more to serve. In reaching the decisions the committee noted that both of them had been contrite and cooperative, and had insight into their professional conduct. None of their actions were done out of malice, and both had otherwise unblemished records (in Ms Christou's case, 26 years). Peter's mother, Tracey Connelly, was 'a skilled and manipulative liar', and there were failings by other agencies too. There was also the context of working in Haringey as a whole. This was described as 'to say the least, a challenging environment', with staff shortages, excessive caseloads and lack of managerial support and supervision. The professional verdict, then, did take account of circumstances and offered some respite from the organisational and public blaming that the social workers had to endure.

Conclusion

This chapter has explored the issue of social workers' responsibility for sad outcomes on their cases. It has taken child protection work as an example, but the same issues arise in other fields of social work too – the multiple meanings of responsibility, the wide, potentially contradictory range of responsibilities, and the nature of individual responsibility in wider organisational, professional and social contexts.

The quotation below, from the book by Dingwall *et al.* discussed earlier in the chapter, captures the debates and dilemmas. Although it refers to child protection work, it could be about any aspect of social work. It is a cool, intellectual look at the challenges, and it is unlikely that it would be well received in an angry press conference or a public inquiry – it would probably come across as a bit too uncaring and calculating. Nevertheless, it is a thought-provoking challenge to populist criticisms of social workers, and to the 'more procedures' response to sad outcomes. It epitomizes the debates about legal provisions, ethical principles and the purposes of social work:

> Child protection raises complex moral and political issues which have no one right technical solution. Practitioners are asked to solve problems every day that philosophers have argued about for the last two thousand years and will probably debate for the next two thousand . . . These difficulties, however, are not a justification for avoiding judgements . . . What matters is that we should not disguise this and pretend it is all a matter of finding better checklists or new models of psychopathology – technical fixes when the proper decision is a decision about what constitutes a good society. How many children should be allowed to perish in order to defend the autonomy of families and the basis of the liberal state? How much freedom is a child's life worth?
>
> (Dingwall *et al.*, 1983: 244)

Questions for reflection

* Do you agree with the quotation from Dingwall *et al.* (1983)? To what extent are child abuse deaths a sign of the social worker's failings (as an individual), social work failings (as a profession), or an inevitable consequence of the legal and societal balances and constraints?

* Do you think it is fair to compare child safeguarding work to driving an ambulance with faulty brakes? In what ways? And what are the consequences of that for social workers' responsibility?

* Think about your experiences in work or on placement, when you have faced a conflict of responsibilities. What or who was it between? How did you deal with it? What values and principles underlie the dilemma and your response?

Useful websites and further reading

The College of Social Work: www.collegeofsocialwork.org/

British Association of Social Workers (BASW): www.basw.co.uk/

General Social Care Council (GSCC): www.gscc.org.uk

Questions and cases

Health and Care Professions Council:

www.hcpc-uk.org/

You may enjoy reading the series of articles by Hollis and Howe, and Macdonald, a classic debate about moral responsibility in social work, and the book by Dingwall *et al.*, a classic analysis of child protection work. They certainly repay reading, but remember that they are old now and the legal and policy detail is long out of date. Look for the underlying issues, which are as pertinent as ever.

10 Crime, punishment and protection

Should the punishment fit the crime? How?

In August 2011 in England, there was a series of violent and destructive riots in a number of cities and towns across the country. Buildings were damaged, in the worst cases completely burnt down, shops were looted, bystanders and local residents were terrorised, and five people were killed (RCVP, 2011). The events received extensive media coverage, shocking people deeply. It is worth remembering that most places were not directly affected, and the huge majority of the population had nothing at all to do with the riots. Most of those who were caught up in the events did not behave criminally, and many showed great courage, care for others and dignity. The country did not descend into anarchy. Law and social order did prevail. But in the state of shock and fear, there were public and political calls for swift and harsh punishments for the rioters, and beyond that for a revival of moral standards.

The Prime Minister, David Cameron, made a speech in which he spoke of mending our 'broken society', using the riots as a justification for many policies that were already on his political agenda. These included 'tougher, no-nonsense policing', higher standards of behaviour in schools, firmer action against troublesome families, a greater sense of community responsibility and more voluntary action, a greater sense of individual responsibility through tackling welfare dependency, challenging human rights legislation which (he claimed) had had a 'corrosive influence on behaviour and morality', and even reforming health and safety legislation which had 'eroded people's willingness to act according to common sense' (Cameron, 2011).

Many of the arguments about the causes of crime echo those about the causes of child abuse and neglect, discussed in Chapter 8: how much is it a consequence of people's individual choices, or of

Chapter 8

culture, family or outlook, or of poverty and circumstances? The aim of this chapter is not to repeat those discussions, but rather to consider the issues of punishment, reform and public protection. How is it best to deal with people who have broken the law, to prevent them re-offending, to rehabilitate them into society, to deter others, and to protect others?

In England and Wales, the responsibility for working with adult offenders in the criminal courts, prisoners and offenders serving sentences in the community, is with the probation service, not social work agencies. However, social workers do work in the youth justice system, as members of youth offending teams (YOTs). Work with offenders was one of the routes through which social work developed as a profession in the late nineteenth and early twentieth centuries, and until 1997 probation officers undertook the same qualifying-level courses as social workers, even though the probation service itself was separate from local authority social services departments (the situation was different in Scotland, where probation services had earlier been transferred to local authority social work departments, where they remain). Nowadays in England and Wales, the probation service and the prison service are part of the National Offender Management Service (NOMS), and probation officers are also known as 'offender managers'.

Although social workers do not usually carry the responsibility for supervising adult offenders in the community, many social workers will (at least from time to time) work with people involved in the criminal justice system – maybe the parents of children on child protection plans or in care, or care leavers, or people who also have mental health problems. Social workers are also likely to work with people who are the victims of crime, notably children who have been abused, adults who have suffered

Chapter 2

domestic violence, or vulnerable adults who have been ill-treated by others in the community (the victimisation of people with learning disabilities is a very disturbing feature, as already shown in Chapter 2, Box 2.3; and see JCHR, 2008; Fyson and Kitson, 2010; EHRC, 2011a).

There are many reasons, then, why social workers need to be aware of criminal law as a context for aspects of their work, and alert to key debates and developments in that field.

The dilemmas of punishment

The general notion of 'punishment' has a number of distinct elements, notably retribution, deterrence, reform, protection and reparation. The Criminal Justice Act 2003 sets these out as 'five purposes of sentencing', and the criminal courts have to weigh these up, taking account of various sentencing guidelines, when deciding what sort of punishment to impose.

Box 10.1: The purposes of sentencing

The Criminal Justice Act 2003, s. 142, gives five purposes of sentencing. Criminal courts have to weigh these up when deciding what sentence to impose:

- *Punishment of offenders.*
  Here, the word 'punishment' is being used in a narrow sense, to refer to the notion of retribution, sentencing the offender according to their 'just deserts'. There is also an element of denunciation, expressing society's disapproval of the crime. The focus is on weighing up the seriousness of the offence, the harm caused and the specific circumstances to give a 'punishment that fits the crime'.

- *Reduction of crime (including its reduction by deterrence).*
  This includes individual deterrence (to prevent the person from re-offending) and general deterrence (to deter others from committing a similar offence).

- *Reform and rehabilitation of offenders.*
  This is aimed at reforming the offender and changing their behaviour, and so links with the purpose of reducing crime. It may include requiring them to attend courses or activities, for example to deal with drug or alcohol addictions.

- *Protection of the public.*
  This may be achieved by removing an offender from society (putting them in prison), restricting their activities (a curfew) or supervising them (probation, and possibly the use of multi-agency public protection arrangements).

- *Reparation by offenders to persons affected by their offences.*
  This may be achieved by paying compensation or through restorative justice.

Young offenders

- Courts and professionals with criminal justice responsibilities for children and young people are required to have regard to the 'principal aim' of the youth justice system, which is to prevent offending by children and young people (s. 37 of the Crime and Disorder Act 1998).

- All courts must have regard to the welfare of a child or young person brought before them (s. 44 of the Children and Young Persons Act 1933), so the youth courts have to balance this with the principal aim of preventing offending.

- It is also proposed that youth courts will have to have regard to a list of the purposes of sentencing that matches the list for adults, shown above. However, the list as given in the Criminal Justice and Immigration Act 2008 did not specify deterrence as one of the purposes. There are differing views about the impact of deterrence on young people (SAP, 2008: esp. 15–18), but protests that it had not been included led to a delay in implementation. The government has said that it will introduce an amendment to confirm that an element of deterrence can be included in sentences for young offenders.

The truth about the five purposes of sentencing is that they all have important parts to play, but simply listing them does not show what to do in any specific case or how to strike the balance between them. The aims of deterrence, reform, protection and reparation may be incompatible with those of retribution (punishment in the narrow sense), which are to give a sentence that fits the crime, a 'just deserts' approach (for a good overview of the issues, see Tonry, 2011).

We shall discuss each of these dilemmas in turn, but even before we get to that, there are difficulties with the term 'just deserts'. As we saw in Chapter 2, there is great disagreement about what is just. Does justice demand the same treatment for someone who is poorly educated and living in poverty, and someone who has had a privileged life? How should the punishment 'fit the crime'? Some people might speak approvingly about the old principle of 'an eye for an eye', but this could not be upheld literally in a modern democratic country. The principle is about proportionate punishment. But what factors should be taken into consideration, and which not?

Chapter 2

Sentencing guidelines

Sentencing guidelines come from three sources. First, Acts of Parliament set the parameters of possible sentences, such as the maximum sentence that can be imposed for a particular offence, and in some cases a mandatory minimum. Notably, legislation prescribes that the sentence for murder shall be life imprisonment (life sentences can be given for other serious crimes too). There are no exceptions to the rule that 'murder means life', even though there are enormous differences between different cases – from a horrific attack to an act of 'mercy killing', from a planned deed to an out-of-character reaction to an unexpected event. In fact, few convicted murderers spend the rest of their lives in prison. The court will set a minimum term, or tariff, that must be served in custody. After this has been served, the prisoner's case will be referred to the parole board to consider their suitability for release. If and when this is granted, they will be released on licence, which lasts for the rest of their life. If they breach the terms of the licence they may be recalled to prison.

The fact that Parliament is involved reminds us that criminal justice and sentencing policy is intensely political. Politicians are always mindful of their public audience, and especially the political importance of being seen to be 'tough on crime, tough on the causes of crime' (the famous New Labour slogan). This gives rise to two more tensions. First, prisons are expensive, and the prison population in England and Wales, at over 85,000, is a huge financial cost. In the current economic situation, it would make good sense to reduce it, and a green paper from the Ministry of Justice in autumn 2010 proposed a number of ways of doing so (MoJ, 2010). However, the political importance of keeping up a 'tough on crime' rhetoric meant that many of these were subsequently vetoed or watered down (MoJ, 2011a; Travis, 2011). Second, the people who are on the receiving end of the toughness are usually from the poorer, most deprived sections of the community. This is likely to provoke more mistrust and unrest than to reduce it: as one of the 2011 rioters is quoted as saying, 'I nick a radio and the world comes down on me, bankers take a million and nothing happens' (RCVP, 2011: 67).

The second source of guidance on sentencing decisions is the Court of Appeal, which gives judgments on appealed cases that indicate to the lower courts the approach that should be applied to specific categories of offence (such as handling stolen goods) and/or offender (such as offenders with serious illnesses).

Third, there is a body known as the Sentencing Council (since 2010; before that, there was the Sentencing Guidelines Council and the Sentencing Advisory Panel). The council issues guidelines that courts must follow. The aim is to ensure consistency and promote public confidence in the criminal justice system. There are guidelines on sentences for certain types of offences (e.g. burglary, fraud, causing death by driving, assault, attempted murder), and on general principles (e.g. sentencing young people, cases of domestic violence, assaults on children, weighing the seriousness of an offence).

The sentencing guidelines are meant to help the court decide on the nature and seriousness of the offence, taking account of the specific facts of the case. They then offer a range of possible sentences, and a suggested starting point. The court can go up or down from the starting point, in the light of aggravating and mitigating factors. In the case of cruelty to a child, for example, aggravating factors that would point to a higher sentence include sadistic behaviour, threats to prevent the child reporting the offence, and failure to seek medical help. Mitigating factors that would point to a less severe sentence include the offender suffering from depression or other mental illness, lack of support, or being dominated by an abusive partner (SGC, 2008). If the court considers that the circumstances warrant it, they have the power to go above or below the suggested range, but cannot go beyond a statutory limit (see the Sentencing Council website, http://sentencingcouncil.judiciary.gov.uk).

Deterrence and just deserts

There can be tensions between the goals of deterrence and a punishment that fits the crime. A relatively minor offence will merit a relatively light sentence, but that may be ineffective in terms of deterrence (a more severe sentence might work better for that). On the other hand, a long term of imprisonment would not be a proportionate response to most offences.

The question of deterrence and just deserts came to the fore in the aftermath of the 2011 riots, when the courts imposed far harsher sentences than would normally have been imposed for certain offences. The Prime Minister encouraged this, to send out a tough message to deter future riots. Examples that hit the news headlines were of a young man sentenced to six months' imprisonment for taking a box of bottled water worth £3.50 from a supermarket, a young single mother who was not at the riots but was sentenced to six months in prison for accepting a pair of looted shorts from a friend, and two young men who were sentenced to four years custody each (upheld by the Court of Appeal) for using Facebook to incite a riot, even though no-one turned up, not even the men themselves (Baggini, 2011).

But does deterrence really work? It implies that offenders are making rational choices, weighing up the possible benefits and costs before deciding whether or not to commit the crime. In reality, many crimes are committed impulsively, or in anger, or carelessly, without any weighing up at all. Some people may think about the possible sentence if they are caught, but it is more likely that they simply weigh up the chances of being caught, and hope to get away with it. More likely still, there is not even that level of premeditation. Many crimes are committed on the spur of the moment, and that seems to have applied to many of those involved in the 2011 riots: as one of them said, 'It was a moment of madness – I regret it every day' (RCVP, 2011: 67; see also the *Guardian* and LSE *Reading the Riots* website). People can be easily influenced and can sometimes get swept away by events, and behave irrationally. Fear of the consequences would not have stopped them then, and a harsh sentence now may have contrary effects, by actually making them more likely to commit future offences. That leads on to the next dilemma.

Reform and just deserts

There are tensions between the goal of rehabilitating an offender, and the notion of proportionate punishment. For example, the chances of reform may be undermined by a prison sentence, which might increase the risk of re-offending. This could be because the offender loses their job or their accommodation, or does not get the help they need to deal with a drug or alcohol problem, which they might have got if they had received a community sentence. It could also be because the person ends up learning more about new ways of committing crime than new ways of keeping within the law. People who have served short sentences (less than six months) – in other words, relatively minor offenders – have higher reconviction rates than those sentenced to longer terms of imprisonment (MoJ, 2010), suggesting that imprisonment has not helped their rehabilitation. Prison has been called a university of crime, and (famously, in a white paper from a Conservative government) 'an expensive way of making bad people worse' (Home Office, 1990: 6).

Misgivings about the negative effects of imprisonment and its high costs lie behind efforts to increase the use of alternatives, such as fines, community sentences and restorative justice. Indeed, some radicals would extend the misgivings from prison to other stages in the criminal justice system, and even into welfare systems. They would point out that most young people who get into trouble with the law eventually grow out of their offending. Life events like getting a partner, getting a job, having a child, all help people to stop criminal behaviour far more effectively than the activities of the criminal justice system or welfare professionals. The best response might arguably be to intervene as little as possible, to minimise the damage that intervention can cause by labelling young people as criminals, reducing their chances of getting a job and desisting from crime. This radical non-intervention approach challenges the over-intrusiveness of reformist approaches, under which disproportionate sentences might be given in the interests of helping the offender (for a riveting exploration of the possible dangerous consequences, see Anthony Burgess' 1962 novel *A Clockwork Orange*). (Just deserts approaches are also critical of over-intervention, but they do not support non-intervention – they support punishments that fit the crime.)

The danger of non-intervention is that it is likely to leave poor people at greater risk of suffering from crime. Poorer communities suffer from more crime than wealthier areas. This is reflected in the findings of the interim report on the 2011 riots. Of the 66 areas where riots occcured, 30 were in the top 25 per cent of most deprived areas of England; furthermore, 55 per cent of the riots took place in the 10 per cent worst areas for vulnerability to long-term unemployment. Nearly 60 per cent of the riots took place in areas ranked in the worst 10 per cent for crime, and over 70 per cent in the worst 10 per cent of areas for social cohesion (RCVP, 2011: 60-2). These figures suggest that intervention needs to be targeted at wider social factors, notably on education and employment, as well as on individuals and families. It takes us on to consider the relationship between public protection and punishment.

Public protection and just deserts

There are two sides to the public protection dimension, both high-profile issues for politicians. There is the priority to keep communities safe from anti-social behaviour and low-level crime, such as unruliness, harassment, vandalism and minor thefts. On a just deserts basis, these may not warrant a criminal sanction, or only a relatively light one; but there is no doubt that they cause great unhappiness to many people, and are likely to continue if no action is taken, or inadequate action. At the other end of the spectrum are the most serious violent and sexual offences. Here, even though an offender might receive a lengthy prison sentence, there may be a risk that they will still be a danger to society following release. Should they be detained for longer than just deserts alone would merit?

The drive to tackle anti-social behaviour was one of the defining themes of the New Labour government of 1997–2010. Much has been written on it, and for a good introduction see Squires (2006, 2008). The Crime and Disorder Act 1998 introduced the anti-social behaviour order, ASBO, to prevent behaviour that was likely to cause 'harassment, alarm or distress'. It could be made in civil courts on the application of local authorities, the police or social housing agencies. Later the grounds for making an ASBO were extended so that it could be made by criminal courts, after a person had been convicted of an offence (with no necessary connection between the matter on which they were convicted and the topic of the ASBO). Breach of an ASBO is a criminal offence and could lead to imprisonment for up to five years. The coalition government proposes to replace ASBOs with two new measures, criminal behaviour orders and crime prevention injunctions. The name may change but the challenges remain the same: how best to protect communities, tolerate different ways of life and reform troublesome individuals.

As for the most serious cases, the concern about public safety led to the introduction of an indeterminate sentence of imprisonment for public protection (IPP), under the Criminal Justice Act 2003 (implemented in 2005). (The equivalent sentence for young offenders was known as an indeterminate sentence of detention for public protection, DPP.) These sentences were used for sexual and violent offences which did not warrant a life sentence, but the offender was considered dangerous and likely to re-offend. The court would set a minimum term that had to be served in prison, but the offender would not necessarily be released after this. They would have to satisfy the parole board that they were safe to be released on licence.

IPPs were very controversial, because they meant that an offender might be kept in prison long beyond their tariff date, without any end in sight, and possibly without any help to change (e.g. see PRT, 2007). They were used much more than had been anticipated, and it was hard for offenders to satisfy the criteria for release, thus adding to the high number of people in prison. On 31 March 2011, there were 8,100 adult prisoners serving life sentences in England and Wales, and 6,550 serving IPPs. Of the latter, more than half, 3,500, were past their tariff date (MoJ, 2011b). Under the Legal Aid, Sentencing and Punishment of Offenders Bill (going through Parliament in winter 2011–12), the coalition government proposed that IPPs would be replaced by a tougher framework of determinate extended sentences and greater use of life sentences. Whatever the changes of law and policy, the challenges of balancing just deserts, fairness for offenders and public safety will remain as contentious as ever. Later in the chapter there is more about policies and issues of protecting the public after offenders have been released.

Reparation and just deserts

The fifth element of sentencing is reparation, making amends to the victim. Restorative justice has become a well-known means of doing this, particularly (but not exclusively) for young offenders. It takes a variety of forms and involves a wide range of practices (see Sherman and Strang, 2007, for a useful overview of research findings). A well-known definition comes from Marshall (1999: 5), who describes it as a problem-solving approach to crime, 'whereby parties with a stake in a specific offence collectively resolve how to deal with the aftermath of the offence and its implications for the future'.

Typically it involves a meeting between the offender and the victim, usually with a facilitator, and perhaps with their family and friends or others affected by the crime; but indirect processes can also be used, such as messages via a mediator or letters. It can be used in schools, communities and as part of the criminal justice system. In the latter, it can be used at various stages: as a diversion from prosecution, before sentencing or after sentence. It is necessary that the offender admits their guilt before the meeting. The meeting gives the victim a chance to say how the offence affected them, and the offender a chance to start making amends. Sherman and Strang (2007) conclude from their review that face-to-face meetings can substantially reduce repeat offending for some types of crime and offenders, notably more serious offences (which is striking, given that restorative justice is more likely to be used for relatively minor crimes). They also found that studies almost always show a high level of satisfaction from victims, with reductions in their levels of anger and anxiety.

However, there are tensions between restorative approaches and just deserts. Restorative justice could, potentially, lead to disproportionate and inconsistent outcomes for different offenders. For example, some victims might demand an excessive payback, whilst others might be satisfied with an apology, for similar offences. For a debate for and against restorative justice, see Cunneen and Hoyle (2010).

The ethics of punishment

Kantians and utilitarians have very different views about the balance between retribution, deterrence, reform, public protection and reparation. The Kantian perspective, with its categorical rules, can sometimes seem very harsh – if stealing bottled water is wrong then it's always wrong, no matter what the circumstances – but on the other hand there is the theme of treating people as ends in themselves, not only as a means to an end. Therefore a Kantian would be very reluctant to punish a person for more than their crime is strictly worth, whether this is to reform the individual, deter others or protect the public. All of these would be treating the offender as a means, not as an end. (Note, however, that the wording of the categorical imperative is ambiguous – 'never as a means *only*' may permit a person to be treated as a means to an end in some respects.) A key point for Kantians is that holding people responsible for their actions is the proper way of treating them with due respect, as individuals in their own right.

Utilitarians would be more open to the idea of sentencing a person for more than just deserts, but also for deterrence, reform or public safety. If the pain inflicted on the individual is outweighed by the benefits to society as a whole, then it would be justified. Pushed to its logical extreme, utilitarianism could even allow for an innocent person to be imprisoned, although Mill tries to balance his utlitarianism with his belief in liberty, as we saw in Chapter 4. A utilitarian argument against imprisoning innocent people would be that a society which does this without regard to individual rights is likely to be less happy overall than one that respects individual liberty.

Virtue and care ethics also have contributions to make. The virtue approach, with its focus on good character, would emphasise the importance of reform, of having courses, treatment and support to help offenders change and desist from further crime. It would recognise that people need support and also a sense of belonging, because character is formed in communities. Some offenders will need a great deal of guidance and support, which is where a care ethic could come in (Gregory, 2010).

For all that, there can be no certainty. Support may be put in place, but eventually individuals have to make their own choices, and they have to accept responsibility for them (echoes of the existentialist approach).

The ethics of care are especially relevant to the increasing importance of reparation and restorative justice. This is not in a 'soft' sense of the victim forgiving the offender, but in the sense of restoring relationships that have been damaged by the offence. In the criminal justice system, offences are treated as crimes against society, and so the state takes the case to court, not the individual victim (they may bring a civil action for damages, but that is different from the criminal case). This has some advantages (it prevents the unfairness that different individuals may be more or less forgiving, and it takes the onus of prosecution off the individual), but it does mean that sometimes victims feel misused or overlooked by the system, their interests and needs overwhelmed by the huge machinery of the courts (Christie, 1977). Restorative justice aims to put victims back into the picture, and to help offenders realise the impact that their behaviour has had on other people.

Public protection

As noted earlier, protecting members of the public from dangerous offenders has become a major political concern and a priority for policy makers and practitioners. It lies behind the development of multi-agency public protection arrangements (MAPPA) and multi-agency risk assessment conferences (MARACs). MAPPA focus on managing the risks posed by sexual and violent offenders. MARACs focus on protecting high risk victims of domestic abuse. There are considerable legal and ethical implications, notably in terms of how much members of the public need to know about the offender's past, and how and when this should be disclosed.

MAPPA aim to protect the public, including previous victims, from serious harm by reducing the risk of re-offending. They were established under the Criminal Justice and Court Services Act 2000, and strengthened by the Criminal Justice Act 2003. The lead agencies are the police, probation and prison services. Other agencies that have a statutory duty to cooperate include local authority social care services, primary care trusts, youth offending teams, housing and education authorities.

MAPPA are intended to ensure that the different agencies work together to discharge their own statutory duties in a coordinated manner. The aims are to identify all relevant offenders; complete comprehensive risk assessments; devise, implement and review risk management plans; and focus the available resources in the most effective way (MoJ, 2009b).

There are three categories of offenders and three levels of risk. Category 1 is registered sex offenders, category 2 is (mainly) violent offenders (that is, sentenced to 12 months or more imprisonment) and category 3 is other dangerous offenders (e.g. people who have previously been dealt with under categories 1 or 2, and are still considered to pose a risk).

The three levels of risk are based on the level of inter-agency coordination required. Level 1 is for 'ordinary' cases that can be managed by one lead agency, sharing information with others as appropriate. Level 2 is when the case has to be managed on a more active inter-agency basis, and will involve regular MAPP meetings. Level 3 is for even more demanding cases, the 'critical few' posing high or very high risk. Here, senior staff will be involved to discuss the case, agree the plans and authorise the necessary resources. For further information about MAPPA, see Wood and Kemshall (2007); Kemshall and Wood (2008); Peck (2011).

MARACs are regular meetings of local agencies (typically every fortnight or every month) to exchange information and produce a coordinated safety plan for high-risk victims of domestic abuse. This includes physical, emotional, mental, sexual and financial abuse, as well as stalking and harassment. They were started in Cardiff in 2003, and there are now around 250 MARACs throughout England and Wales (Steel *et al.*, 2011).

The organisation CAADA ('Coordinated Action Against Domestic Abuse') is working with the Home Office to develop MARACs. It has an informative and comprehensive website, including a 'risk identification checklist' for identifying cases where there is a high risk of domestic abuse, stalking and honour-based violence (the CAADA-DASH checklist). There is also useful guidance about MARACs, sharing information with other agencies, and informing the person in danger (CAADA, 2007). It is considered good practice to tell the victim that the meeting is taking place, but their consent is not required and if it is considered unsafe to tell them about it, it is not necessary to do so. The person does not attend the meeting itself, but information can be presented on their behalf by an independent domestic violence adviser. The perpetrator should not be informed about the meeting directly (it is acknowledged that they may get to know about it indirectly), is not invited and should not be told anything about the safety plan.

Third party disclosure

There are guidelines regarding the sharing of information with other agencies and individuals ('third parties') who are not part of MAPPA and MARAC structures. This could be to people such as employers, youth group leaders, church representatives and neighbours. It may be done if it is necessary to prevent serious crime and ensure the safety of others, but the core human rights principles of necessity, fairness and proportionality still apply. Guidance stresses that only the minimum amount of information necessary should be disclosed, only to people who really need to know, and when there is a specific risk of a crime (CAADA, 2007; MoJ, 2009b). A non-specific risk is not enough. The CAADA guidance on MARACs gives an example of a man with convictions for violence against women moving to a new neighbourhood. This would not be disclosable unless he presented a likely risk to a named woman or a particular household. Further, the offender should normally be informed about the plan to disclose, unless this is likely to increase the risk to the victim or others. (Research into the operation of MAPPA has found that the offender often agrees to the disclosure, and may even take part in it: Wood and Kemshall, 2007; Kemshall and Wood, 2008.) The

Chapter 12

implications of these principles are shown in the case of *H and L v A City Council* [2011], discussed in Chapter 12.

Third party disclosure is also contentious because of the risks it may create for some of the offenders. Notably, the concern has been that if information about a child sex offender is given to members of the public, the news may spread and give rise to vigilante attacks and public disorder. Some might say that the offender has lost his right to privacy because of his crime and the risk he presents, and the overriding consideration has to be the safety of the public. If disclosure puts him at risk, so be it. However, things are not as straightforward as that because there is the danger of counter-productive outcomes, where offenders 'go underground', hiding from agencies rather than cooperating with them. This would mean they are not properly monitored and not getting the help they need. Disclosure might have the paradoxical effect of increasing risk to the public.

Under MAPPA and MARACs, the initiative for disclosure lies with the agencies, and they decide who should be told. However, there has been a high-profile campaign for wider disclosure about child sex offenders. This was the campaign for a 'Sarah's law', named after Sarah Payne, a girl who was murdered by a convicted child sex offender in 2000. The title was chosen to echo a US law for public disclosure of details about child sex offenders, 'Megan's law'.

Since 2008 there has been a scheme for members of the public to ask the police for checks to be made about people they think may be a danger to children. This is the Child Sexual Offender Disclosure scheme (Home Office, 2010; Kemshall and Wood, 2010). It was piloted in four police areas from 2008 to 2009, and has since been extended. It has been a nationwide programme since spring 2011. Although anyone can ask for the checks, the information can only be given to a parent or carer. It is not a general disclosure to the wider public, and in that sense it is not a direct equivalent of 'Megan's law' (Home Office, 2010: para. 2.1). A strict warning about confidentiality is given to the people who receive the information, and they have to sign an undertaking to respect it.

The issue of public safety continues to be a live issue, and in winter 2011–12 there was a consultation for a 'Clare's law', to allow an individual to be informed if the person they are in a relationship with has a conviction for domestic violence (Home Office, 2011a).

Conclusion

This chapter has considered the often-contradictory principles of punishment, and the dilemmas of public protection. The latter has covered recent and forthcoming changes regarding anti-social behaviour, extended sentences for serious offenders, monitoring in the community and disclosing information about offenders. The topics of information-sharing and confidentiality are explored further in Chapter 12.

The chapter has highlighted the social and political pressures that shape policies on punishment and public protection. The ethical dilemmas are profound, but often newspaper headlines and politicians' speeches give little room for calm reflection and analysis of the causes of crime and the best responses.

Questions for reflection

- Have you been the victim of a crime? What happened? How did it make you feel at the time, and how do you feel about it now? What did you want to happen to the person who did it?

- Do you think that the names and addresses of convicted child sex offenders should be made available to the general public? Think about children in your family, who you know and love. What do you *really* think?

Useful websites and further reading

Burgess (1962) *A Clockwork Orange*.

Tonry (ed.) (2011) *Why Punish? How Much? A Reader on Punishment*.

Pickford and Dugmore (2102) *Youth Justice and Social Work*, 2nd edition.

Sherman and Strang (2007) *Restorative Justice: The Evidence*.

Sentencing Council: http://sentencingcouncil.judiciary.gov.uk/index.htm. This includes a link to an interactive website called 'You be the judge' (http://ybtj.justice.gov.uk/). This has film of actors playing out a court case, and then questions for the viewer to decide what sentence to give – informative and thought-provoking!

CAADA (Coordinated Action Against Domestic Abuse): www.caada.org.uk

NACRO (National Association for the Care and Rehabilitation of Offenders): www.nacro.org.uk

Howard League for Penal Reform: www.howardleague.org

Prison Reform Trust: www.prisonreformtrust.org.uk

Victim Support: www.victimsupport.org.uk

11 Culture and difference

Can we reconcile cultural diversity and equal standards for all?

As we noted in Chapters 2 and 5, values of anti-discriminatory and anti-oppressive practice are fundamental to social work. Great importance is attached to respecting different cultures and lifestyles, recognising their strengths, not measuring them in negative ways against the norms and practices of the majority. These values are widely promoted in international and national codes of social work ethics and practice (e.g. IFSW and IASSW, 2004; BASW, 2012).

Similar values are reflected in the law. There is the general principle that all people are equal before the law, and human rights apply to all. There is specific legislation to prohibit discrimination and promote equal opportunities, such as the Equality Act 2010 (see Chapter 2). There are also specific provisions to ensure that services are designed and delivered in ways that meet the needs and

wishes of people from different communities – for example, s. 22 of the Children Act 1989, that local authorities must have regard to the race, religion, culture and language of children in care, and the 'respect principle' in the Mental Health Act 1983 Code of Practice (see Box 11.1).

For all that, it sometimes seems that there is a lot more rhetoric than reality in our society about treating all groups equally, and social work does not escape that criticism. There are two main questions:

- Why might social work be oppressive to the very people it is trying to help?

- What happens when there is clash between the values of the majority group, and those of the minority?

This chapter tackles the first of those questions by looking at the ways that people from black and minority ethnic communities (BME) experience mental health services. Discriminatory and unequal treatment of black and minority ethnic people is found throughout society, including public services such as criminal justice, education and social care (EHRC, 2010). This chapter takes mental health services as an example. It highlights the guiding principles of mental health work which set high standards of anti-discriminatory practice, but the reality is that services have often fallen short and failed to meet the needs of BME communities. This raises challenging questions about how effective our values really are in helping us to identify and tackle prejudice and discrimination.

The chapter addresses the second question by discussing the issue of forced marriages. This shows the tensions between modern western values of individual choice and women's rights, and the values of some groups in the United Kingdom about community, kinship and honour. It highlights the limitations of a relativist approach and shows the potential for strengthening this with more radical understandings.

Mental health and difference

It is important to note at the outset that the term 'BME' covers a wide range of people, from African-Caribbean men, who are more likely to be subject to compulsory treatment, to Southeast Asian women who are less likely to receive timely and appropriate services, even when severely unwell (HM Government, 2011: para. 6.20). It also includes Africans, people of Mediterranean origin, Irish people and East Europeans; new migrants and long-settled communities; travellers; asylum seekers and refugees; young people and older people.

For all that diversity, there is a long record of research that shows that people from BME communities in the UK are more likely to experience mental ill health than the white British majority, and less likely to see mental health services as helpful (for summaries see SCMH, 2002; NIMHE, 2003; DH, 2005; Morgan et al., 2006). Some groups, notably African-Caribbean and black African people, are significantly more likely to be subject to compulsory measures to enforce assessment and treatment (NIMHE, 2003: 12–13).

The reasons for these differences are complex and contested. One leading study, known as the AESOP study, found that rates of schizophrenia were nine times higher in the African-Caribbean population than the white British, and six times higher for black Africans (Morgan *et al.*, 2006). It also noted that in the Caribbean the incidence of schizophrenia is similar to that of white British people in the UK. This suggests that the cause is not biological differences (that black people are by nature more likely to develop the condition), but social factors. These might include living in a predominantly white environment, poverty and social discrimination, and different treatment within the mental health services themselves.

The issue of different treatment came to a head with the death of David Bennett in 1998 (Blofield, 2004; for a discussion see Laird, 2010). Mr Bennett was an African-Caribbean man, a Rastafarian, and had a diagnosis of schizophrenia. He died at the age of 38 in the Norvic Clinic, a medium secure psychiatric unit in Norwich, England. Mr Bennett had a long history of mental health problems, with a 'revolving door' pattern of becoming unwell in the community because of not taking his medication, being admitted to hospital, behaving aggressively, being transferred to a secure unit, recovering, and being discharged back to the community.

In October 1998 Mr Bennett was a patient at the Norvic Clinic. One night he and another patient got into a fight about using the telephone. The other patient was racially abusive towards Mr Bennett, but the staff did not challenge the other man about this. They decided that Mr Bennett should be moved to another ward. On hearing this, Mr Bennett became angry and hit a member of staff extremely hard, injuring her badly. There was a struggle to restrain Mr Bennett. He was forced to the ground, face down, and a number of staff lay on top of him to hold him there. He was kept like that for nearly half an hour, as a result of which he suffered cardiac and respiratory failure and died. To put it baldly, he was crushed to death.

Mr Bennett's sister, Dr Joanne Bennett, campaigned hard over several years for a thorough inquiry into what had happened. This was eventually set up in 2003, and reported in 2004 (Blofield, 2004). The inquiry looked at the history of Mr Bennett's case, as well as the events of the night. It found that although there was no deliberate racism from staff, there had been no proper attention over the years to his ethnic, cultural and religious needs. As individuals, staff at times treated him kindly, but at other times 'as a nuisance who had to be contained' (Blofield, 2004: 12). He was subject to notably high levels of anti-psychotic medication.

The inquiry concluded that Mr Bennett's experience was unlikely to have been different from that of other BME patients with similar mental health problems, and that this could be attributed to 'institutional racism'. This concept had come to prominence in the inquiry into the racist murder of Stephen Lawrence, the young black man who was killed in 1993. After a long campaign by his parents, an official inquiry was established in 1998, reporting in 1999 (Macpherson, 1999). The term refers to the unconscious attitudes, stereotyping and everyday practices that systematically disadvantage minority ethnic people. The important point is that it is not deliberate, knowing discrimination, but unthinking assumptions and routine behaviour.

Following the David Bennett inquiry, the government launched a programme called *Delivering Race Equality in Mental Health Care* (DRE: DH, 2005). It was an ambitious programme, with a wide range of goals to improve services. Two of the goals were to reduce the disproportionate rate of admission of people from BME communities to psychiatric inpatient units, and to reduce the disproportionate rates of compulsory detention. The programme lasted five years. The end-of-programme review concluded that there had been little change in either of these (NMHDU, 2010: 37–8).

The Mental Health Act 1983

The Mental Health Act 1983, as amended by the Mental Health Act 2007, is the principal piece of legislation in England and Wales that governs the treatment of people with 'mental disorder'. This term includes conditions such as depression, schizophrenia, obsessive compulsive disorders, post-traumatic stress disorder, dementia, personality disorders and eating disorders (DH, 2008b: para 3.3). It also includes learning disabilities, but a person with a learning disability and no other mental disorder cannot be compulsorily detained for treatment unless their disability is associated with abnormally aggressive or seriously irresponsible conduct (Mental Health Act 1983, s. 3; see also DH, 2008b: paras 3.13–15 and Chapter 34).

Most people who need mental health services receive them on a voluntary basis, in the community. Even when people need to be treated in hospital, the majority are admitted informally (i.e. with their consent). The Mental Health Act 1983 contains provisions under which people may be subject to interventions by professionals when they do not consent, in the interests of their own health or safety, or the protection of the public. It specifies the grounds for formal (compulsory) admission to hospital, either for assessment (ss. 2 and 4) or for treatment (s. 3), and for emergency detention of a person already in hospital (s. 5). It also has provision for guardianship of patients in the community (s.7, when a minimum level of supervision is necessary), and for supervised treatment outside hospital (s. 17A, community treatment orders).

Overriding people's consent has to be balanced with proper safeguards, and the aim of the 2007 Act was to adjust this balance to take account of the many changes since 1983, notably the increase in community care, changing knowledge and attitudes about mental health, and the impact of human rights legislation. But as we have noted before, Acts of Parliament are political creations, and the history of the 2007 changes shows that there was also a high level of concern to strengthen the public protection aspects. In particular, this was driven by media coverage of a small number of cases where people with mental health problems had killed members of the public. The first bill, published in 2002, attracted widespread opposition from mental health professionals and service users, and led to the creation of the Mental Health Alliance, a coalition of organisations to resist the proposals. The government eventually withdrew that bill, and after a period of consultation published another in 2004. This was also opposed and later withdrawn, so the 2007 Act was the third attempt – an indication of how hard it is to get the legal framework right for such demanding decisions about individual freedom, welfare and public safety.

There is a Code of Practice for the Mental Health Act. The fourth edition of this was published in 2008, to go with the amended Act (DH, 2008b). Agencies and practitioners have to 'have regard' to it, and there must be 'sufficiently convincing justification' for any departure from it (DH, 2008b: para. iv). The new Code introduced five guiding principles, shown in Box 11.1. Respect for different backgrounds is one of them. The Code also says:

> Care must always be taken to avoid diagnosing, or failing to diagnose, mental disorder on the basis of preconceptions about people or failure to appreciate cultural and social differences. What may be indicative of mental disorder in one person, given their background and individual circumstances, may be nothing of the sort in another person.
>
> Difference should not be confused with disorder. No-one may be considered to be mentally disordered solely because of their political, religious or cultural beliefs, values or opinions, unless there are proper clinical grounds to believe that they are the symptoms or manifestations of a disability or disorder of the mind. The same is true of a person's involvement, or likely involvement, in illegal, anti-social or 'immoral' behaviour. Beliefs, behaviours or actions which do not result from a disorder or disability of the mind are not a basis for compulsory measures under the Act, even if they appear unusual or cause other people alarm, distress or danger.
>
> (DH, 2008b: paras 3.5 and 3.6)

Box 11.1: Mental Health Act 1983 Code of Practice: five guiding principles

Purpose principle

Decisions under the Act must be taken with a view to minimising the undesirable effects of mental disorder, by maximising the safety and wellbeing (mental and physical) of patients, promoting their recovery and protecting other people from harm.

Least restriction principle

People taking action without a patient's consent must attempt to keep to a minimum the restrictions they impose on the patient's liberty, having regard to the purpose for which the restrictions are imposed.

Respect principle

People taking decisions under the Act must recognise and respect the diverse needs, values and circumstances of each patient, including their race, religion, culture, gender, age, sexual orientation and any disability. They must consider the patient's views, wishes and feelings (whether expressed at the time or in advance), so far as they are reasonably ascertainable, and

---

follow those wishes wherever practicable and consistent with the purpose of the decision. There must be no unlawful discrimination.

Participation principle

Patients must be given the opportunity to be involved, as far as is practicable in the circumstances, in planning, developing and reviewing their own treatment and care to help ensure that it is delivered in a way that is as appropriate and effective for them as possible. The involvement of carers, family members and other people who have an interest in the patient's welfare should be encouraged (unless there are particular reasons to the contrary) and their views taken seriously.

Effectiveness, efficiency and equity principle

People taking decisions under the Act must seek to use the resources available to them and to patients in the most effective, efficient and equitable way, to meet the needs of patients and achieve the purpose for which the decision was taken.

(DH, 2008b: paras 1.2–1.6)

The implications for ethics and social work

The summary of the mental health legislation has highlighted the importance of anti-discriminatory principles, but the experiences of BME service users and the limited impact of the DRE programme, as described above, suggest that there is a wide gap between the principles and the reality. What are the implications for social work?

Mental health social workers usually work in multi-disciplinary teams, alongside members of other professional groups, especially doctors, nurses, psychologists and psychiatrists. They work in a variety of settings, including hospitals, day centres and community-based services, notably as members of community mental health teams (CMHTs), or child and adolescent mental health services (CAMHS). After additional training and approval, they may take on the role of approved mental health professional (AMHP) (Mental Health Act 1883, s. 13). This role was created by the amendments under the Mental Health Act 2007, replacing that of 'approved social worker'. A wider range of professionals may now undertake this work, but all must undertake specialist training (see NIMHE, 2008; GSCC, 2010c).

A key part of the job of mental health social workers is to put the social perspective on mental health, if necessary to assert it against the dominant medical models. They are required to promote the rights and dignity of service users, to enable them to participate in decision-making as far as possible, and to challenge discrimination in all its forms. These tasks are not unique to social workers (they are in the Code of Practice, and are part of the requirements for all AMHPs, whatever their professional background), but there may be tensions between this approach and the understandings, attitudes and practices of other professional groups.

The big challenge to social work values comes from the notion of institutional racism. We can widen this concept and speak of institutional discrimination, because similar issues arise in other areas too, notably the treatment of learning disabled people and older people – unconscious attitudes, stereotyping and routine practices that sweep away proper respect for individuals' dignity and rights (e.g. Mencap, 2007, 2012; JCHR, 2008; and the cases of Winterbourne View and Steven Neary, discussed in Chapter 13).

The concept of institutional discrimination raises serious challenges for all of the major ethical approaches. It challenges the idea that care is enough, because, as the David Bennett inquiry found, most of the staff were caring, most of the time. They did not commit deliberate ill-treatment, but even so he was treated unfairly and, at the end, badly. It challenges the idea that individual virtue is enough, because again, most of the staff meant well. It challenges utilitarianism, because it shows how easily the welfare of the individual is lost under the great pressures to protect the majority. And it challenges Kantianism, because it shows how hard it is for individual rationality to identify what really needs to be done and ensure it is put into effect. Even categorical moral duties can be overwhelmed by the rules, roles and routines of organisational life. This analysis reminds us that none of the four ethical approaches is comprehensive, flexible and robust enough by itself to deal well with all matters. We need to keep them all in play, to support and to challenge each other.

What about the different approaches to freedom? The libertarian approach challenges the high rates of compulsory detention, making us ask whether these steps are really necessary, but carries two serious risks. The first is that it brings very high thresholds for state intervention, which might prevent people getting the help and protection they need early enough; but second, once they have passed the threshold, it tends to make coercive and harsh responses more likely. The existentialist approach draws attention to the importance of individual freedom, but this is hard to apply to some of the most severe cases, where people are seriously unwell and need intervention for their own safety.

The relativist and radical approaches seem to be most relevant to the question of mental health and BME communities, but they are not straightforward and there can sometimes be tension between the values of tolerating different lifestyles and those of ensuring safety of individuals and equality of treatment. A relativist approach emphasises the importance of cultural differences, but this has to underpin the provision of appropriate services, not be used to minimise people's needs or deny individuals their rights ('it's their culture' as an excuse for inaction). A radical approach would focus on the wider economic and structural context of mental ill health, and the way that people from some communities are more likely to be labelled as mentally unwell. It would argue for services that address those circumstances, along with wider action for political and organisational change, but it must not lose sight of individuals' choices and needs, including sometimes the need for immediate protective action.

Forced marriages

The tensions between relativism and radicalism can be seen in sharp profile by looking at law and ethics in regard to forced marriages. This has become a prominent issue in the United Kingdom and other western countries in recent years, leading in England to the Forced Marriages (Civil Protection) Act 2007. This came into force in November 2008. For reviews of the progress of the Act, see MoJ (2009c) and Home Affairs Select Committee (2011).

The dominant public image of forced marriage is of young women from South Asian communities, notably Pakistan and Bangladesh, but it is not confined to those countries, nor to women. It also occurs in communities from East Asia, the Middle East, Africa and Europe, and in gypsy and traveller communities. Men can also be forced into marriage, and people with learning disabilities are especially vulnerable (HM Government, 2010d).

In England and Wales there is, currently, no specific crime of 'forcing someone to marry', although there is in Scotland, the Forced Marriage (Protection and Jurisdiction) (Scotland) Act 2011, which came into force in November 2011. Legislation to make it an offence has been proposed (e.g. Home Affairs Select Committee, 2011) and became the subject of a Home Office-led public consultation in December 2011 (Home Office, 2011b). Many of the actions associated with it are crimes, such as abduction, false imprisonment, assault, rape and murder, and perpetrators can be prosecuted for them. The idea of introducing a specific criminal offence is controversial (see Gill, 2011). Supporters argue that it would send a strong message about the unacceptability of the practice, and would give victims stronger grounds on which to negotiate with their families. Against this, opponents consider that it might be tokenistic, but might also make reconciliation less likely (Gill, 2011).

Under the Forced Marriages (Civil Protection) Act 2007, courts in England and Wales can issue a forced marriage protection order. This is a type of injunction to try to prevent a forced marriage. It can impose requirements such as ordering a person to hand over passports and birth certificates, to stop intimidation and violence, to reveal the whereabouts of a person, and to enable a person to return to the UK. Breach of an order is not in itself a criminal offence (although the action may be) but is contempt of court and could be punished by up to two years in prison (MoJ, 2009c: 15).

There is a government Forced Marriage Unit (FMU), established in 2005. This is run jointly by the Foreign and Commonwealth Office and the Home Office. It acts in individual cases, offers advice and training, and produces statutory guidance (HM Government, 2008a) and practice guidelines (HM Government, 2009a, 2010d). The FMU also seeks to increase public and professional understanding of the issue. It has a comprehensive website with an online training course.

According to the Ministry of Justice report on the first year of the Act, the FMU dealt with 1,600 reports of possible forced marriage in that year, leading to 420 active cases and 86 protection orders (MoJ, 2009c: 3, 12). By February 2011, a total of 293 orders had been made (Home Affairs Select Committee, 2011: para 8).

The FMU documents and training materials are unequivocal about the unacceptability of forced marriage. They hold that it is a violation of human rights and unacceptable in all major religions. They emphasise the difference between forced marriage and arranged marriage. The latter is acceptable, as long as both people are genuinely free to choose whether or not to go ahead with the marriage. This is a well-established distinction, although in reality things may not always be as simple as that. An-Na'im (2000), for example, holds that it is better seen as a continuum. At the ends the differences between forced and arranged marriages are clear, but in between there is a considerable grey area, where unspoken pressure, persuasion and coercion are hard to untangle.

The FMU materials give strong messages about the importance of alertness to identify possible cases and determined action to prevent forced marriage. For example, they stress what they call the 'one chance rule', that practitioners might get only one chance to speak to the person and thereby save a life. They also emphasise the dangers of involving families and trying to negotiate with them, because this might lead to the person being quickly silenced or removed from the country. The FMU online training course says that:

> due to the nature of forced marriage and honour-based violence, some of the principles within existing guidance may inadvertently place victims at greater risk of harm. This includes the principle that the best place for a young person is with their family and the practice of attempting to resolve cases through family counselling and mediation. In cases of forced marriage, it's vital that you *do not* initiate, encourage or facilitate family counselling or mediation – whether offered by community councils, religious or professional groups.

(FMU, 2011: emphasis original)

This approach is seen as a particular difficulty for social workers, because it is so different to their usual ways of working (MoJ, 2009c: 22). The issue of whether or not allowance should be made for different cultures is also seen as a potential problem. The FMU advice is given in Box 11.2.

Box 11.2: Culture and forced marriage

The Forced Marriage Unit online training course (FMU, 2011) asks whether the following statement is true or false: 'When dealing with cases of forced marriage it's important to make allowances for different cultures'.

The correct answer, according to the FMU, is false. The text reads:

> Yes, this statement is absolutely false. It's important to understand the motives that drive parents to force their children to marry, but these motives shouldn't be accepted as justification for denying them the right to choose a marriage partner and enter freely into marriage. Forced marriage is a violation of children's rights under the UN Convention on

---

the Rights of the Child (UNCRC) as well as a form of violence against women and an abuse of human rights. However, professionals should always seek to establish the facts of a case to avoid making any preconceived judgements.

What do you think about this answer?

Some of the crimes that are committed to force a person to get married, or to punish them for refusing, are horrific. They certainly cannot be justified on the grounds that 'it's our culture' (or excused on the grounds of 'it's their culture') just as violence cannot be justified on that basis in any community. Even so, it is worth asking whether the FMU's strident tone is the most effective approach.

One of the things that the MoJ first year report noted was that there was a need to engage better with the more closed black, Asian and minority ethnic communities, 'to encourage them to hear and respond to the messages enshrined in the Act about respect for individual choice' (MoJ, 2009c: 6). Perhaps it is not surprising that there is resistance, given the dogmatic tone of the FMU materials, with their message that the communities cannot be trusted and must be corrected. This tone of suspicion and superiority is likely to alienate communities that are already anxious about their survival, turning them inwards and reinforcing the practices that the outsiders are trying to change (An-Na'im, 2000).

In a blistering article, Sherene Razack (2004) challenges the assumptions that lie behind the standard western approaches to forced marriages, particularly in Muslim communities. It is important to say that she is not defending forced marriages or the violence that can sometimes be associated with them. On the contrary, she is clear that it is vital to challenge male violence towards women in all communities. She would agree with the FMU that cultural justifications are unacceptable, but her reasoning is very different. She does not want to descend into 'cultural deficit' models ('they are patriarchal and uncivilised'), and she also wants to challenge the growth of ever more suspicious and stigmatising approaches to Muslim communities. She writes:

> The policing of Muslim communities in the name of gender equality is now a globally organised phenomenon and one that has become even more pronounced after the events of September 11, 2001 . . . The policing is organised under the logic that there is an irreconcilable culture clash between the West and Islam . . . They are tribal and stuck in pre-modernity, the argument goes, possessing neither a commitment to human rights, women's rights nor to democracy. It is the West's obligation to defend itself from these values and to assist Muslims into modernity, by force if necessary, as the wars in Afghanistan and Iraq both underline. The body of the Muslim woman, a body fixed in the Western imaginary as confined, mutilated, and sometimes murdered in the name of culture, serves to reinforce the threat that the Muslim man is said to pose to the West and is used to justify the extraordinary measures of violence and surveillance required to discipline him and Muslim communities.
>
> (Razack, 2004: 129–30)

Razack holds that western (mis-)understandings rest on three stereotypes: the civilised European, the imperilled Muslim woman and the dangerous Muslim man. Razack argues for a deeper understanding, based on a radical analysis rather than one that focuses on cultural differences. The radical analysis would highlight the difficult circumstances of immigration, especially the laws and practices that keep families apart, and the experiences of hardship and racism in the new countries that drive communities into themselves. For Razack, the key is to understand Muslim communities in context. The lazy stereotyping and the emphasis on culture mask the economic circumstances and the impact of racism:

> Acknowledging little or no responsibility for the conditions in which Muslim migrants in the West live, and indulging in the fantasy of a superior nation who must discipline and instruct culturally inferior peoples, Western states pursue policies of surveillance and control that heighten the level of racism those communities experience and that exacerbate the conditions under which Muslim communities become even more patriarchal and violent towards women.
>
> (Razack, 2004: 132)

For Razack, arranged and forced marriages alike spring from an impulse to control women's sexuality, and it is almost inevitable that such controls will be used more vigorously when communities feel themselves threatened and isolated. Razack argues that the way forward is to pay more attention to the effects of sexism and racism. Focusing on cultural difference runs the risk of stereotyping and alienating the whole community (and thereby still leaving women in danger). Instead, the focus should be on tackling sexism within Muslim (and non-Muslim) communities, and on tackling racism. This includes institutional racism in the agencies involved. The concern should not only be to end familial violence against women (although of course that must remain, with a wider range of services and support) but also to end the violence of poverty, limited opportunities, discrimination and oppressive immigration and asylum legislation (Razack, 2004: 166–9).

Social work values and social change

Tackling social inequalities and promoting diversity have become much-used catchphrases in social work, often used together, as though they are natural partners. However, the topic of forced marriages shows that they are not always easily compatible. Tackling the oppression of women and girls may lead to conflict with some ethnic communities.

How best then can we promote the values we believe in without being oppressive and imperialist, imposing the norms of the dominant culture on minorities? An-Na'im (1994) suggests a relativist way forward. He holds that ' efforts to articulate shared values must be founded on mutual respect and sensitivity to the integrity of other cultures, especially in view of colonial and post-colonial power relations between the North and South' (An-Na'im, 1994: 68). He offers two guiding strategies, internal discourse and cross-cultural dialogue. Outsiders must not impose their own values but can influence a situation through:

- engaging in their own internal discourse [i.e. role modelling, by working for change in their own communities];

- supporting the right of internal participants to challenge prevailing perceptions whilst avoiding overt interference . . .;

- engaging in cross-cultural dialogue to exchange insights and strategies of internal discourse . . .;

- highlighting moral and philosophical commonalities of human cultures.

(An-Na'im, 1994: 68).

This may be a wise approach, but it is a slow and uncertain one. Social workers are likely to come across people who need help *now*, urgently. The challenge is to reconcile the gradual, community perspective with the protection of individuals.

Razack's radical approach adds an extra dimension. It means addressing the ways that a community's values and behaviour are affected by external factors, notably social, economic and legal discrimination (e.g. immigration laws). This wider, radical and campaigning role may not suit all social workers, and how far one can pursue it as part of one's paid job will be limited by the type of organisation one works for (Banks, 1999), but nevertheless social work has often held that one of its core duties is to challenge wider social inequalities (e.g. IFSW and IASSW, 2004; BASW, 2012).

History offers a warning for social work on this point, about its capacity to stand up to wider societal prejudice and institutional discrimination. Our values and ethical codes may not be strong enough to resist. Lorenz (1994) shows how this happened in Nazi Germany, as social workers used their key skills, such as assessment, advice and support giving, to carry out tasks for the oppressive regime. This is not to pass facile judgments on people who were living through terrifying times, but to make the point that social work skills can be used for good or ill. For Lorenz (1994: 68) this is a sign of 'the weak connection between methods and values in social work', and we certainly do not have to go back as far as 1930s Germany to find evidence of that (see, for example, the swingeing critique of current UK social work by Preston-Shoot, 2010 and 2011). It is a warning to be careful about how much we claim for social work values, and to be vigilant to the ways that social work can, inadvertently, add to discrimination and oppression.

Conclusion

This chapter has explored the dilemmas of how to value difference and ensure safety and equality, by looking at the topics of BME communities and mental health, and forced marriages. Both of these examples bring out the importance of seeing individuals and families in their wider social context, to understand different rates of mental ill-health and to the importance given to arranged marriages.

The discussion has brought out the strengths and limitations of relativist and radical approaches. Relativists focus on the cultural context, and radicals the economic and structural contexts, although of course there are overlaps between them. As usual, it is important to keep both sides in the equation, using the strengths of one to counteract the limitations of the other. For both, it is important not to lose sight of the needs and rights of individuals. The challenges are that the values of toleration can sometimes be in tension with equality and safety; there are the dangers of slipping into cultural deficit thinking; and there are powerful social and organisational forces at play (notably racism, sexism, inter-professional dynamics, law and politics), making change very hard to achieve. All of this shows why social work values of respecting difference and treating people equally are much discussed but often so difficult in practice. That is not to say social workers should give in: on the contrary, it makes it more important than ever to keep thinking and working, in ways that are resolute and realistic.

Questions for reflection

- An-Na'im (1994) exemplifies a relativist approach, with his strategies for helping to achieve cultural change in other communities. How might you apply them in practice?

- Razack (2004) exemplifies a radical approach, with her argument that to end forced marriage we should concentrate less on culture and more on tackling sexism and racism. How might you put these principles into practice?

- Can you square these two approaches?

- Think back to the discussion about racial discrimination in mental health services. Why do you think it has proved so hard to reduce the disproportionate rates of admission to hospital and compulsory detention? What are the implications for social work?

- Do you think that Lorenz (1994) is right to say that there is a weak connection between methods and values in social work? How could it be strengthened?

Useful websites and further reading

Mind: www.mind.org.uk

Rethink: www.rethink.org

Forced Marriage Unit: www.fco.gov.uk/en/travel-and-living-abroad/when-things-go-wrong/forced-marriage

BBC Ethics website on forced marriage: www.bbc.co.uk/ethics/forcedmarriage/

Razack (2004) 'Imperilled Muslim women, dangerous Muslim men and civilised Europeans: legal and social responses to forced marriages'.

Bogg (2010) *Values and Ethics in Mental Health Practice.*

Sewell (2009) *Working with Ethnicity, Race and Culture in Mental Health: A Handbook for Practitioners.*

Thompson (2011) *Promoting Equality: Working with Diversity and Difference*, 3rd edition.

12 Confidentiality, information-sharing and openness

> *What are the limits of confidentiality? What sort of information can be shared, when, and to whom?*

Confidentiality, information-sharing and openness are important principles for social work, but the tensions between them raise many challenging questions. We have already discussed some of the dilemmas in Chapter 10 when we explored the pressures for and against disclosure of information about potentially dangerous people to third parties, such as neighbours and parents. In this chapter we take a closer look at the ethical, social and legal dimensions and demands.

Chapter 10

There are ethical and legal requirements to respect confidentiality of information, but also to share it for service users' well-being and protection. There are regular calls for more effective information-sharing, driven by the demands of inter-professional and inter-agency working and the pressures of an increasingly risk-averse society. These are countered by pressures to preserve individuals' privacy and not to use personal data beyond the purposes for which it was collected. Furthermore, there are demands to open up decision-making processes in areas which have traditionally been confidential, notably courts that deal with welfare matters, such as the family courts and the Court of Protection. Supporters of these campaigns argue that wider knowledge will ensure fairer treatment for the individuals and families going through the courts, and increase public confidence in the processes. Opponents argue that it will hinder sensitive treatment for the most vulnerable families, and unfairly expose them to public curiosity and criticism.

For most social workers, certainly those working for local authorities in the UK, there are limits to the confidentiality that they can promise to service users. If there are serious concerns about the safety of children or vulnerable adults, then the law and their ethical duties point them towards disclosing this to other relevant agencies and professionals. But this soon starts to raise difficult questions: how serious do the concerns have to be to warrant disclosure? If the service user does not agree to disclosure, when should that be overridden – and how, legally and ethically? Who should information be shared with – only other professionals, or individuals who are directly affected, or even more widely, with the general public? And whose interests does confidentiality really serve – the service users' or the professionals'?

The chapter explores the dilemmas in four stages. First, it shows the ambiguity of the ethical arguments, which point in different directions, and the gaps that can sometimes arise between expressed principles and actual practice. Second, it considers the fast-moving and contentious social context, where there are hotly contested arguments about individuals' rights to privacy *and* to information. Third, it outlines the legal context and summarises government guidance for sharing information lawfully. Finally it investigates the pressures for and against opening up the family courts to media reporting, which sharply raise the question of whose interests confidentiality really serves.

The ethical context

Confidentiality is one of the traditional values of social work, appearing in social work ethical codes around the world (e.g. IFSW and IASSW, 2004; BASW, 2012; for discussion, see Clark, 2006b; Swain, 2006; Banks, 2012). At first sight it would seem to be a good example of a categorical, Kantian value. Confidentiality is a categorical duty because it respects the autonomy of the service user, recognising their right to privacy and control over their own lives, treating them as ends in themselves. Kantians believe in the importance of telling the truth and keeping promises, so if one has promised to keep a confidence, then one must, regardless of the consequences.

In reality, the duties of confidentiality are soon qualified, to allow the possibility of disclosure in cases of serious risk to the service user or others. This can be seen as a consequentialist, utilitarian argument against confidentiality – one should break it if the greater good is served by doing so. Even so, one should not forget the Kantian message, because it warns us against promising confidentiality too easily (we must be honest about the limits) and about overriding it too readily. As Munro (2007) argues, a strong concept of confidentiality is an important protective barrier to defend individuals from excessive intrusion by the state.

In fact, the ethical context is complex and it is not as simple as saying that Kantians are for confidentiality and consequentialists against. It is possible to argue for confidentiality on consequentialist grounds – for example, that it is necessary for a trusting professional relationship, and trust is important because it means that service users are more likely to be forthcoming and honest, which means they can be helped more effectively. Confidentiality brings better results. The importance of trusting relationships also chimes with the ethics of care; but on the other hand, the care approach would also be prepared to break confidentiality in the interests of the cared-for person. Virtue ethics is ambiguous too. The virtuous person will behave with discretion, respecting confidences but also knowing when and what to share with others.

Information-sharing is the other side of the coin, and again there are ethical arguments for and against. From a utilitarian point of view, sharing knowledge about risks can ensure the greatest good for the greatest number by protecting people from harm; but on the other hand, sharing information too freely might undermine important social values and leave us in a less happy society overall. From a care point of view, it can ensure that people get the most suitable help, but it might destroy trusting relationships. The virtuous person shares what is necessary in the interests of the service user and wider society, but the challenge is to know what the mid-point is between indiscretion and reticence. The Kantian believes in telling the truth, so would allow sharing of information (but no more than necessary) provided that one has been honest with service users from the outset about the limits of confidentiality.

This notion of being honest with service users from the start is often seen as a fundamental principle, but McLaren (2007) shows that even so, social workers do not always do it. The main reasons they give are that they think it will stop service users being open with them, or that it will make the professional relationship more difficult. McLaren argues that forewarning is essential to ensure that service users are not deceived. It should be built into agency procedures, and accompanied by assurances about what advice and support the service user could expect if information is to be disclosed.

In summary, ethics offers no absolute answers about the merits of confidentiality or information-sharing. Decisions have to be made in the circumstances of each individual case, within a framework of trying to balance competing imperatives. Honesty about this is a vital starting point. The theme of getting the right balance on a case by case basis is also crucial to the legal approach, discussed later in the chapter.

The social context

Issues of confidentiality and information-sharing are explored thoroughly in Clark and McGhee (2008), *Private and Confidential? Handling Personal Information in the Social and Health Services*. In particular, the book draws attention to the wider social context which shapes the way these matters are addressed in health and social care.

In the introduction to the book Clark and McGhee describe the traditional understanding of confidentiality in terms of three layers. First is the individual to whom the information refers; second is the front-line worker who gathers that information, and who has a responsibility to handle it trustworthily; and third are other professionals and agencies, who may wish or need to know the information. In the traditional model, the individual owns the information that relates to him or her, and it should only be spread further with their agreement, or if doing so is considered necessary for their own well-being or that of others. In the conclusion, Clark and McGhee argue that this is no longer a realistic model (and see Clark, 2006b; Swain, 2006). They identify four trends in society that are challenging and changing the traditional model.

First is the increasing complexity of the ways that health and social care are delivered, usually through inter-agency working and often by teams of workers rather than the old model of one worker taking the lead. The reality is a highly permeable, porous working environment, with information being shared within and across agencies and professions all the time. Doing so is an important part of delivering a high-quality service (e.g. so that other workers know what to do if a colleague is unavailable), but can easily be disrupted by differences of agency priorities and professional cultures (Richardson and Asthana, 2006).

Second, there is the huge growth of information and communication technology (ICT) for recording, storing, transmitting and sharing information. This increases the potential benefits and risks of gathering, storing and exchanging all manner of communications and data. Parton (2009) gives an important analysis of the impact of ICT on social work policy and day-to-day practice. He argues that it has contributed to a shift of focus, away from relationships and in-depth understanding of people's lives, to one of gathering, sharing and monitoring information. This is not an entirely new trend (the rise of procedural and managerial control of social work has been long noted – e.g. Howe, 1992), but the pace has quickened since the mid-1990s as new technologies have been introduced.

For Parton (2009), ICT is changing the nature and form of *knowledge* in social work, moving it to 'a database way of thinking'. Social workers become primarily information processors, and the relational and social dimensions of the job are diminished. In theory, the work becomes more ordered, transparent and accountable, but in reality there are a number of drawbacks. One is that the database mentality gives an illusion of certainty that the realities of social work practice and service users' lives do not justify. Furthermore, the database becomes the focus of attention, a virtual reality, rather than the 'real reality' of people's lives. As well as those things, the fact is that the systems often don't work very well. Information gets lost, they can break down, it is easy to make mistakes, and the amount of information can become overwhelming. The problem that lies behind social work tragedies is, nowadays, not so much a shortage of information, or a failure to pass it on, but rather that the information was there but was not understood properly, not recognised for what it was (see Reder and Duncan, 2003, discussing this with regard to the Victoria Climbié inquiry). The database mentality breaks information down into its different parts, but what is important is to understand it as a whole. This needs well-trained and skilled professionals with a 'communication mindset' (Reder and Duncan, 2003) that keeps them alert to the dangers of misunderstanding.

Clark and McGhee's (2008) third point is about social attitudes to privacy. These are changing and ambiguous, with blurred boundaries about what is acceptable or not. An example is the intrusive media coverage of celebrities' lives. At times the public seems to enjoy the salacious stories about footballers, actors, politicians and the like, but at others it deplores the journalistic tactics that gets them (as in the *News of the World* telephone hacking scandal of 2011). The courts sometimes uphold legal action by the celebrities to 'gag' the press, but in other cases allow publication. Another example of public ambivalence is the behaviour of individuals on the internet. There is some conduct that is exceptionally self-revealing, and some that is highly exploitative of others, but there are also calls for tighter regulation and privacy controls. These ambivalent attitudes are reflected in the debates about media reporting of the welfare courts, discussed below.

Fourth, Clark and McGhee (2008) identify the rise of citizens' rights movements and service users' campaigns, which have pursued questions about how personal information is shared and used, challenging professionals' ways of doing things. Once more, there are tensions for social work that reflect the variety of public opinion. Some argue for greater privacy rights for individuals and tighter rules on handling personal information, others for greater openness from organisations about their policies and decisions. This can extend to demands to know more about the information the agencies hold on individuals, and more about the way that cases are dealt with in the courts.

The legal context

The legal context has three dimensions: legislation on data protection and freedom of information, the common law and human rights law. The websites of the Information Commissioner's Office and the Campaign for Freedom of Information are invaluable sources of guidance about data protection and information-sharing.

The Data Protection Act 1998 is an example of UK law that is shaped by the European Union. It was passed in order to bring the 1995 European Data Protection Directive into force in the UK. It was implemented in 2000. Schedule 1 of the Act sets out eight data protection principles, which it takes from the European Directive. The first is that personal data must be processed fairly and lawfully. 'Personal data' is information about a living individual from which that person can be identified. It includes (amongst other things) social work and health records, whether electronic or on paper. 'Processed' is a wide-ranging term that includes collecting, storing, sharing, combining, altering and destroying data. 'Fair' and 'lawful' mainly relate to confidentiality. They mean that the data must be processed with the consent of the person who is the subject of the information, or in pursuit of legal duties, or within legal powers. Personal data must not be used in a way that is incompatible with the purpose for which it was obtained. It must be adequate, relevant and not excessive; accurate and up-to-date; and must be kept only as long as is necessary.

The Freedom of Information Act 2000 came into force in January 2005. It gives individuals the right to request information held by public authorities (e.g. local and central government, hospitals, state schools, the police), but it does not apply to personal data. However, the two Acts are closely inter-connected. If the request is for personal data and is made by the person concerned, it should be dealt with under the Data Protection Act instead. If it is for personal data about another person, there may be restrictions on releasing it if doing so would be a breach of confidentiality.

Common law holds that where there is a confidential relationship, such as doctor–patient, lawyer–client or social worker–service user, the information will normally be treated as confidential. However, there are exceptions to this, such as if the information is already public, the person gives consent to disclosure, or if sharing is in the public interest, notably to prevent serious harm or serious crime.

In terms of human rights law, the ECHR upholds citizens' rights to a private life (Article 8), which requires the state to respect the confidentiality of information given by them or about them. This is a qualified right and interference may be allowed if it is necessary and proportionate (see Chapter 2, especially Box 2.2). It is important to appreciate that these are strict tests. Disclosure must be really necessary ('a pressing need'), limited to only what needs to be disclosed in the specific circumstances, and must be done fairly.

An example of the need for rigorous thinking about whether and how to disclose information is the case of *H and L v A City Council* [2011], mentioned in Chapter 10. In 1993, H had been convicted of a serious sexual offence against a child. He had been imprisoned for it, but had always maintained his innocence. He had a later offence of dishonestly concealing the circumstances of his conviction. He and his partner, L, were active in the disability rights movement, and ran a company to provide consultancy to a number of public bodies and voluntary organisations. In 2009, his local authority was informed of the first conviction and a pending prosecution (on which he was subsequently acquitted). The authority held a meeting, without informing H and L, and decided to inform all the organisations with whom he had contact. The Court of Appeal, with Lord Justice Munby giving the leading judgment, was highly critical of the authority's actions (and of the earlier High Court judgment that had upheld them). The issue was one of proportionality, with a need to balance the protection of children against the right to privacy. There had to be a pressing need to tip the balance towards disclosure, and this did not arise in this case because H's work did not bring him into contact with children. Further, a blanket disclosure was not lawful. There had to be a case by case assessment of the need to disclose, and H and L should have had the opportunity to put their point of view.

Government guidance published in 2008 gives a useful checklist of seven key questions to help decide when disclosure is appropriate. These are shown in Box 12.1.

Box 12.1: Information-sharing: seven key questions

These questions come from HM Government (2008b) *Information Sharing: Guidance for Practitioners and Managers.* The guidance gives detailed information to explain each of them, and what practitioners must do to ensure that they can answer them confidently. The information is summarised here. The strong message is that if in doubt, practitioners should seek advice.

1   *Is there a clear and legitimate purpose for you or your agency to share the information?* For example, is it a normal part of your job, is there a statutory duty or a court order to do so? If no, you should not share. If yes, go on to Question 2.

2   *Does the information enable a living person to be identified?* If no (for example, if it is anonymised), it can be shared. Otherwise, go on to Question 3.

3   *Is the information confidential?* For example, was it provided in the expectation of confidentiality? Information is confidential to the agency as a whole, not to the individual practitioner, but workers still have a duty to preserve confidentiality – for example, only to share information for genuine purposes. If it is not confidential, you may share. Otherwise go on to Question 4.

4   *If the information is confidential, do you have consent to share?* You will have to consider whose consent is required, and whether they are able to give informed consent. You will have to consider issues of competence and capacity (as discussed earlier, in Chapter 7). In some circumstances it may not be appropriate to seek consent, for example if it will place another person at risk. If you have consent, you can share. If not, go on to Question 5.

5   *If consent is refused, or there are good reasons not to seek consent, is there a sufficient public interest reason to share the information?* The key concepts here are necessity and proportionality. If a child or adult is at risk of serious harm, sharing information without consent may be justified. If you do not have sufficient reason, you may not share. If yes, go on to Question 6.

6   *If the decision is to share, are you sharing information appropriately and securely?* For example, only as much information as needs to be shared, accurate and up-to-date, distinguishing between fact and opinion. Go on to Question 7.

7   *Have you properly recorded your information-sharing decision?* Record your decision and the reasons for it. If you did share information, record what and with whom.

Opening up the family courts

Arguments about the reporting of child and family court cases are an intriguing example of the tensions between privacy and openness, and the impact of public pressure. Similar issues arise in response to calls to open up the Court of Protection to media reporting. These were highlighted by the

case of Steven Neary, discussed in Chapter 13. (Court of Protection hearings are usually held in private, but journalists were allowed into Steven's hearing because the case had already been widely reported in the press. The judgment was published using real names, rather than non-distinguishing initials.)

Chapter 13

Traditionally, proceedings involving children have been held in private, but this has led to accusations of unfairness and secrecy. The main impetus for change has been in the field of private law (divorce and separation cases, applications for residence and contact orders), where fathers' rights groups have led high-profile campaigns to draw attention to what they see as the courts' bias against men, in favour of mothers. In the field of public law (care and adoption proceedings), there has been pressure from parents' rights groups concerned about the powers of the state and the dangers of miscarriages of justice.

Such concerns were intensified by a number of high-profile criminal cases in the early years of this century, where parents were convicted of murdering their children on the basis of expert evidence that was later discredited. Two of the most prominent cases were those of Sally Clark, convicted in 1999, whose conviction was quashed in January 2003 after a second appeal, and Angela Cannings, whose 2002 conviction was quashed in December 2003. The media pressure was vital in raising doubts about the evidence. Although these were criminal cases, the campaigns raised concerns that similar injustices might be happening in the care courts. They made the point that expert evidence is not always reliable and full scrutiny is required, but courts do not always seem willing to listen to alternative points of view. The argument was that if this happens in criminal trials that are open to the public, how much more likely are miscarriages of justice in closed hearings, especially civil proceedings where the standard of proof is lower?

The Websters

A high profile case that raised the question of allowing journalists into the family courts arose in 2006. This was the case of the Websters, a couple from Norfolk whose three older children had been the subjects of care proceedings in 2004. The central issue then had been an allegation that one or both of the parents had caused non-accidental fractures to one of the children (known as child B). The parents held that there were medical reasons for the fractures (an inherited condition), but the medical evidence ruled out alternative explanations. The parents continued to assert that they did not cause the injuries. The local authority held that in any event there were other concerns about the standard of care and the parents' willingness and ability to make the necessary changes. The judge made care orders and freeing orders for adoption, and the three children were subsequently adopted.

In 2005, Mrs Webster became pregnant again and her new baby, Brandon, was born in May 2006. Shortly before he was born, the parents fled to Ireland because they were afraid that he would be taken into care, but they returned to England later. There was extensive media coverage of the case, but when the local authority started care proceedings, the court made an order imposing very strict reporting restrictions. The Websters appealed against this with the assistance of two media organisations (the BBC and Associated Newspapers Limited). The appeal was heard by Mr Justice Munby in October 2006: *Re Brandon Webster, Norfolk County Council v Webster and others (No 1)* [2006].

The judgment highlights the difficult balancing act that has to be undertaken (para. 80). The parents have rights under Articles 8 and 10 of the ECHR to tell their side of the story, but Articles 8 and 10 are qualified rights, and may be restricted in the wider interests of (amongst other things) 'the rights and freedoms of others' (see Chapter 2). The parents also have rights under Article 6 to a fair trial, which in their opinion would have been aided by press coverage of the proceedings. The child has rights under Articles 6 and 8, and the children's guardian argued that for him these pointed towards privacy of the proceedings. The local authority could argue that it has Article 10 rights to put its side of the story (it was happy for the release of anonymised judgments from the care proceedings, in the hope that this would counter the criticisms of the way it had handled the case, but did not want reporters to attend the hearings). The media may wish to assert that they have Article 10 rights to receive and impart information (but these are qualified rights). The witnesses and others involved have Article 8 rights to privacy (but again, these are qualified rights, especially as regards the professionals). Then there are the wider public interests of preserving freedom of expression *and* confidentiality, and in ensuring that justice is done and confidence in the courts is maintained.

Chapter 2

The judge held that the reporting restrictions should be lifted. He identified four factors that tipped the balance: that there was an allegation of a miscarriage of justice, that the parents themselves wanted the publicity, that there had already been extensive publicity, and that it was important for the full facts to emerge in a way that commanded public confidence (para. 99 of the judgment).

The agreed plan in the care proceedings on Brandon was that he and his parents should go to a residential placement. This went well, and later Brandon went to live at home with his parents. In the course of the proceedings, the Websters' new lawyers got permission to seek fresh expert opinions on the injuries to child B. An expert from the USA identified the cause as scurvy (*Re Webster (A Minor)* [2007]). Further medical reports were obtained from professors of paediatric nutrition and paediatric radiology, who agreed that this was highly likely. In summer 2007, Brandon's case came to final hearing. By agreement, it ended with no order and Brandon staying at home (*Norfolk County Council v The Parents & BC (By His Child's Guardian)* [2007]). At the same hearing, Mr and Mrs Webster indicated that they intended to appeal against the care orders on their other children.

Their application for permission to appeal was heard in December 2008, and judgment given in February 2009 (*Webster (The Parents) v Norfolk County Council & Others (Rev 1)* [2009]: see paras 52–8 for an account of the medical reports). The court refused them leave to appeal. The two main reasons were that the medical evidence could and should have been obtained at the time (para. 180), and that there was no point in re-opening the care hearing because the adoption orders could not be overturned (para. 178). The main points here are that adoption orders are absolute and final (a categorical argument); and also, if they could be overturned this would be likely to reduce the number of people who apply to adopt (para. 146: a public policy, consequentialist argument).

There was great sympathy for Mr and Mrs Webster, and recognition that there may have been a miscarriage of justice. However, there was nothing that could be done. The judge commented that mistakes will occur in any system operated by human beings, but said he was satisfied that everybody involved had acted in good faith (para. 193). Social workers who are so used to being heavily criticised by the courts and the media might find this a surprisingly sanguine view. The judge also said that it was 'idle to pretend' that having journalists in court would have made any difference (para. 198).

Policy developments

The pressures for and against openness of family proceedings have been reflected in a chain of policy announcements. In 2006, the government issued a consultation document on ways of improving transparency *and* privacy in family courts (DCA, 2006c). This proposed that the media should be allowed into the family courts as of right, although any reports that they wrote should be anonymised. The consultation responses showed a clear split between media organisations which supported the proposals, and organisations representing children and court professionals which disagreed (DCA, 2007b). The government then revised its proposals, saying that journalists would not be allowed in as of right. Instead, it proposed that there should be better information about cases involving children, including making anonymised family court judgments (or summaries of them) publicly available, and better information for the people involved (MoJ, 2007).

However, pressure for media attendance continued and in 2008 another government policy document changed the story again (*Family Justice in View*, MoJ, 2008b; for a summary of the developments see Fairbairn and Gheera, 2009). This announced that the media would now be allowed to attend family proceedings, although the court would have the power to restrict attendance and what was reported. Since April 2009 it has been possible for accredited journalists to attend child and family cases. Also, a pilot project ran from November 2009 to December 2010 in five family courts, to publish anonymised transcripts of all judgments (MoJ, 2011c). These are available on the BAILII website (www.bailii.org.uk). The significant thing about them is that they are 'ordinary' cases, not the complex or controversial ones that get to the higher courts. The report on the pilot scheme found that there was concern for the privacy of the families involved (MoJ, 2011c). At the time of writing it is not certain whether the pilot will be extended.

As regards media attendance, misgivings about its impact remain. The Children's Commissioner for England (2010), in a study of children and young people's views, found considerable anxiety about what and how much they would feel able to disclose to professionals if they thought a journalist would get to find out about it. Most of the children and young people did not want any information to appear in the public arena.

Furthermore, a High Court judgment in 2011 found that a care case had been inaccurately reported in a leading national newspaper, using dramatic language that clearly implied criticism of the agencies for over-reacting, by a journalist who had not attended any of the hearings (*Re L (A Child: Media Reporting)* [2011]). No doubt it will seem very odd to most social workers that the attendance of journalists is being held up as a way of sharing trustworthy information with the public, about what child care social work and care proceedings really involve.

Conclusion

This chapter has discussed the considerable tensions that exist between the duties of confidentiality, information-sharing and openness. It has shown how these reflect complex, often uncertain and contradictory ethical principles, social priorities and legal requirements. It has also reviewed the arguments for and against greater openness and reporting of the family courts. There is concern about this from some viewpoints, and grounds for scepticism. On the other hand, good journalism can increase public knowledge and understanding, and can uncover wrongdoing and cover-ups. The

persistence of courageous individuals is also important (notable examples are David Bennett's sister, mentioned in Chapter 11, and the parents of Stephen Lawrence). Further examples of the way that individuals and the press can expose ill-treatment and injustice are discussed in the following chapter (Winterbourne View and Steven Neary).

In terms of the major ethical approaches, and in terms of human rights, the challenge is that neither confidentiality nor sharing is automatically on top. They have to be weighed against one another in the whole context of each case, and against other key values, such as the rights to life, freedom from inhuman and degrading treatment, a fair hearing and private and family life. It is important to appreciate that whatever the decision, it will have implications beyond the individuals directly involved. Fundamental social values are at stake, notably privacy, protection, proportionality and fairness.

Questions for reflection

- Would you always explain about the limits of confidentiality to service users, at the start of your working relationship with them? What are your reasons, for or against?

- Swain (2006) questions whether it even makes sense to talk of confidentiality as a core social work value, given that it has so many limitations. Instead, he argues that we should replace it with 'an honest and explicit acknowledgement that confidentiality cannot be guaranteed, but that client information will be treated with respect' (Swain, 2006: 93). Do you agree? What are the advantages and possible drawbacks?

- Who do you think was responsible for what happened to the Websters? The judge was careful not to criticise anyone, but what do you think about that? Should someone be blamed?

- List the arguments for and against journalists attending care hearings. Do you support it? What would you say about it to parents or children and young people involved in care proceedings?

Useful websites and further reading

DfE information-sharing webpage: www.education.gov.uk/childrenandyoungpeople/strategy/integratedworking/a0072915/information-sharing

HM Government (2008b) *Information Sharing: Guidance for Practitioners and Managers*, via the DfE information-sharing webpage.

HM Government (2009b) *Information Sharing: Further Guidance on Legal Issues*, via the DfE information-sharing webpage.

Information Commissioner's Office: www.ico.gov.uk

Campaign for Freedom of Information: www.cfoi.org.uk

Clark and McGhee (eds) (2008) *Private and Confidential: Handling Personal Information in the Social and Health Services*.

13 Organisations and individuals

What is the nature of individual responsibility in organisational contexts?

This chapter considers issues of individual conduct and responsibility in organisational settings. All organisations face the demands of getting the work done, managing within budgets, balancing the needs of different service users, and being sensitive to the needs of staff. All organisations have their own cultures and routines, their established ways of doing things. All organisations are made up of different people, with likes and dislikes, conflicts and alliances. Some members of the organisation are powerful by virtue of their position (e.g. senior managers), and others because of personal characteristics (e.g. a great deal of experience, a sharp tongue, or physically intimidating). Where does individual responsibility fit into this?

Questions about the relationship between individual responsibility and organisational context arise in four particularly challenging areas:

- *Poor professional practice* (e.g. a worker not carrying out their tasks, not being reliable, not making sound decisions). There is a responsibility on the organisation to help the worker improve, but in the interests of service users, managers may have to take competency proceedings against the worker. What should a worker do if they think that a colleague is not performing well, or if they think the organisation condones poor standards?

- *Criminal conduct* (e.g. theft from a service user, fraud, ill treatment of a service user). Clearly an organisation should not tolerate this, but unfortunately there are examples of appalling treatment of service users, and of organisational cultures that do not challenge it. What should a worker do if they find themselves in such a situation?

- *'Professional boundary' transgressions* (e.g. inappropriate personal relationships with service users). Some behaviour is clearly unacceptable, but many boundary issues are uncertain and shadowy (Doel *et al.*, 2009, discussed later in this chapter). How do personal conduct, professional roles and organisational responsibilities interact?

- *Resource restraints* (e.g. the organisation withholding or withdrawing services on financial grounds). What should a social worker do if they see that resource limitations are causing service users to suffer, or if they disagree with how their organisation proposes to use limited resources?

Social work ethics makes hard demands on social workers to balance individual and organisational responsibilities. The BASW code of ethics, for example, calls on social workers to strive to carry out the stated aims of their employers provided that they are consistent with the code, but also to work to change policies and procedures that do not meet professional standards (BASW, 2012). The code emphasises the corresponding duties on employers to have systems and approaches that enable social workers to comply with the code. It also states explicitly that social workers 'should be prepared to report bad practice using all available channels including complaints procedures and if necessary use public interest disclosure legislation and whistleblowing guidelines' (BASW, 2012: para. 3.9).

Whistleblowing

Whistleblowing is the term used for raising a concern about work with managers, approved regulators, or other external bodies, including the media. Ethical and legal duties to raise concerns about mal-practice have to be balanced against ethical and legal duties to respect confidentiality of information about individuals, and employees' duties to follow the policies and procedures of their organisation. The purpose of the Public Interest Disclosure Act 1998 (PIDA) is to give a framework for such balances and protect workers who raise genuine concerns about possible criminal offences, failure to fulfil legal obligations, miscarriages of justice, health and safety dangers and cover-ups. More than that, it was meant to encourage organisations to develop their own policies and procedures, and promote a culture in which it is acceptable for staff to voice their concerns, so that problems are nipped in the bud (CSPL, 2005; Bowers *et al.*, 2007: esp. 385–407).

The PIDA 1998 specifies three categories of protected disclosure, shown in Box 13.1. There are different thresholds for different types of disclosure. Whistleblowing to (say) a newspaper requires a higher standard of certainty and seriousness than raising the matter with one's employer, if it is to be protected under the Act.

Box 13.1: Public Interest Disclosure Act 1998

The PIDA 1998 amended the Employment Rights Act 1996, and came into force in July 1999. If a worker makes a disclosure that is protected under the Act, but then suffers victimisation or dismissal, the Act allows them to bring a claim for compensation in an employment tribunal. Note that the Act does not cover students on courses run by educational establishments such as universities (Employment Rights Act 1996 s. 43K(1)(d)); however, social work courses are required to have effective whistleblowing procedures: GSCC (2002b).

The three categories of protected disclosure under PIDA 1998 are:

1 *Internal disclosure*
   This is reporting the concerns to a manager or director. The disclosure will be protected if the whistleblower makes it in good faith (e.g. not maliciously), and they have reasonable cause to believe that the information tends to show that the malpractice has occurred, is occurring or is likely to occur.

2 *Regulatory disclosure*
   This is reporting the concerns to a regulatory body, such as the Care Quality Commission. The disclosure is protected if it meets the same grounds as an internal disclosure, *plus* the whistleblower reasonably believes that the matter is substantially true and is relevant to the regulator.

3 *Wider disclosure*
   This is reporting the concerns to wider audiences such as the police, the media or service user groups. It is protected on the same basis as a regulatory disclosure, *plus* if it is not made for personal gain and is reasonable in all the circumstances. One of more of the following four conditions must also apply: (a) that the whistleblower reasonably believed they would be victimised if they raised the matter internally or with a prescribed regulator; or (b) there was no prescribed regulator, and they reasonably believed that the evidence was likely to be concealed or destroyed if they raised it internally; or (c) they had already raised it with the employer or the regulator; or (d) the matter was of an exceptionally serious nature.

For further information about the Act and whistleblowing generally, see the website of Public Concern at Work (PCAW), a registered charity that is the leading campaign and advice group on whistleblowing in the UK: www.pcaw.org.uk

---

The protections of PIDA should really be a last resort. Problems should be dealt with long before things get that far, through a climate in the organisation that facilitates openness, and well-publicised procedures for staff to report concerns confidently, and confidentially if necessary. Despite all this – all the policy announcements, the requirements of ethical codes, the protection of the law, and general public approval for people who blow the whistle on dangerous practice or criminal conduct – it has to be said that drawing attention to a problem is still a difficult and often risky activity for the whistle-blower. It can take a great deal of courage.

The whistleblower might be seen as a hero by the public, but could well be seen as a villain by the organisation and their professional colleagues. A notable example is Margaret Haywood, a nurse who won the *Nursing Standard* 'Patients' Choice' award in 2009 for using secret filming to expose ill-treatment of older patients at the Royal Sussex hospital in Brighton, but who was then struck off the nursing register for breaching patient confidentiality (Edemariam, 2009). Also, being a whistleblower can be a personally difficult and disconcerting experience, provoking feelings of disloyalty and anxiety about the consequences for colleagues, service users and their families. Ward (2008) describes how her involvement in secret filming of how older people were treated in care homes provoked feelings of fear, dishonesty and uncertainty, even though she was sure that she was 'doing the right thing'.

Box 13.2: Principles of responsible whistleblowing

Whistleblowing can be considered a form of advocacy for service users, a way of upholding their interests in the face of malpractice and organisational resistance to change (Greene and Kantambu Latting, 2004). However, as PIDA 1998 makes clear, there is a process that one should normally go through. Going through the proper stages increases the chances of success and minimises the risks to the whistleblower. Drawing on Greene and Kantambu Latting's (2004) checklist for responsible whistleblowing, and guidance on the PCAW website, eight key principles are:

- *Keep calm, and try to weigh up the risks and outcomes before taking action.* What are the risks of taking a particular course of action, or of not acting? Risks to who (e.g. the service user, other workers, yourself)? Who might be the best person to speak to first?

- *Obtain advice.* There may be a specific member of staff who advises on these issues. Local authority children's services in England are required to have such a post, known as the Local Authority Designated Officer (LADO). Other options are the team manager, a trusted colleague, a professional body such as BASW, a trade union, and PCAW.

- *Remember that there may be an innocent explanation.* Do you feel able to discuss the issue with the colleagues about whom you are concerned? If not, why not? More information might shed new light on the situation, or may bring support for change. However, this needs

---

careful thought. It would not be appropriate if the concern is about something that might be a crime, or if the whistleblower fears he/she would be victimised. Again, the important thing is to seek advice.

- *Establish a track record of credibility.* Newer members of staff will need to take extra care to have good evidence for their claims.

- *Do not assume that others in the organisation do not care.* Others may already have concerns, and be ready to support you.

- *Keep careful records,* such as a chronology of what happened and who said what. You are not a detective, but a clear and accurate picture of what happened is crucial.

- *Do not use whistleblowing procedures to pursue complaints or personal grievances.* There should be other procedures for such matters. Be sure to keep your objectivity.

- *Use the chain of command.* Unless the situation is extreme, respect the organisation's line management structure, and work up it as far as necessary.

Ill treatment of service users

It is not unusual for internal whistleblowing to be ignored or denied (PCAW, 2011, found that this happened initially to 40 per cent of cases in the care sector). Even disclosures to regulators may not be acted upon. That was what happened to Terry Bryan, a senior nurse who tried to raise concerns in 2010 about the ill treatment of patients at Winterbourne View, a private hospital near Bristol for people with learning disabilities and autism. It was run by an organisation called the Castlebeck Group, which had twelve mental health hospitals (including Winterbourne View) and twelve adult social care facilities registered with Care Quality Commission in England (CQC, 2011).

Mr Bryan wrote to his employers about his concerns in October 2010, but nothing happened. He then tried to alert the CQC, but even though he contacted them three times, there was no response. In fact, the CQC had inspected Winterbourne View three times in the previous two years, but had not found anything untoward. Mr Bryan then went to the BBC, which employed an undercover journalist to get a job as a support worker at the hospital. He secretly filmed what he saw. The film was shown on *Panorama* on BBC1 in May 2011, and provoked a national outcry. It showed a culture of abuse, with staff deliberately inflicting pain on the patients. There were acts of routine violence, insults and assaults, bullying and victimisation. Force was used when not necessary, for 'punishments' and at times, it seemed, simply for the entertainment of the staff. The hospital was subsequently closed down by the CQC. Serious failings were found in over half of Castlebeck's establishments (CQC, 2011). In particular, staff were inadequately trained and supervised.

Nursing and care work seem to generate especially disturbing stories of neglect and ill treatment by staff (see also EHRC, 2011b, on shortcomings in home care services). There is a range of factors behind this. The public expectations of nurses and care workers make the behaviour particularly shocking – after all, they are paid to provide care. Then there is the nature of the work, which legitimately involves touching and sometimes restraint, so the social and psychological barriers against physical contact are already weakened. Other factors are the physical and mental vulnerabilities of older people, people with learning disabilities and people with mental health problems, and the social stigma that these groups suffer, which again lowers the normal taboos about such conduct. On top of all that, staff are often poorly paid, trained and supported; and patients or service users may be isolated and without regular visitors to check how they are, whether in residential care or their own homes.

As social workers we should not be complacent. The GSCC website gives details of cases where social workers have been suspended or struck off the social care register for breaking the social care code of practice. There are, regrettably, cases of social workers stealing from service users, defrauding their employers, falsifying case records, and having inappropriate, sometimes sexual, relationships with service users or members of service users' families (GSCC conduct hearings web pages; and see GSCC, 2008; Banks, 2010; McLaughlin, 2010).

Of course, the vast majority of social workers behave perfectly properly. It is only a very small number whose behaviour has led to hearings before the GSCC conduct committee. The GSCC reported 278 cases where misconduct was proved between 2006 and the end of September 2011 (GSCC, 2011a), out of a registered workforce of over 100,000 social workers and social work students. Of the proven cases, fifty-three (about a fifth) involved inappropriate relationships with service users.

Professional boundaries

Concern about the number of cases involving inappropriate relationships had been raised by the GSCC in 2008, and led them to commission two research studies into professional boundaries: Doel *et al.* (2009, 2010) and Parker (2009). In November 2011 the GSCC published guidance for social workers on professional boundaries (GSCC, 2011b). The concept does not only include the limits of professional conduct *in* work, but also what behaviour is appropriate or inappropriate *outside* work. Some behaviour might raise grave questions about the individual's suitability to be a professional social worker, and also risk undermining public confidence in the profession as a whole.

One of the key points made by Doel *et al.* (2009: 76) is that the boundaries of acceptable behaviour are more like an area of overlaps and shadows, rather than a clear line or wall. Some behaviour is clearly unacceptable (stealing from a service user, for example), but many others are much less certain. Doel *et al.* argue against having yet more rules and ever tighter regulations. Their argument is that this approach makes staff fearful and therefore less likely to be open; also, it is impossible to give a list of bullet points that will cover every eventuality, and any transgression is unlikely to be simply because one bullet point was missing. Instead, they called for organisations to promote an atmosphere of 'ethical engagement', where staff are able to discuss these issues, helping them to develop ethical competence.

This is the approach that the GSCC guidance adopts. It states that social workers should not enter into relationships with service users outside their professional role, but rather than giving an exhaustive list of rules it offers case examples and questions for reflection. It gives four useful questions for general guidance (GSCC, 2011b: 7):

- Would you be comfortable discussing all of your actions, and the rationale for those actions, in a supervision session with your manager?

- Would you be uncomfortable about a colleague or your manager observing your behaviour?

- If challenged, could you give an explanation as to how your actions are grounded in social work values?

- Do your actions comply with the relevant policies of your employer?

Box 13.3: Professional boundaries and whistleblowing scenarios

Doel *et al.* (2009, 2010) used a series of case scenarios in their research into what sort of conduct is considered acceptable or unacceptable for welfare professionals, in and outside work. Statements 1–4 in the list below come from their study. The guiding questions here ask you to think about how serious you consider each of the twelve scenarios, and what you would do.

- Do you think the scenarios below are examples of professional misconduct?

- How serious, on a scale of 0 (not at all) to 5 (extremely serious), would you rate each of them? What factors affect your answer?

- Would you report such situations if you became aware of them? Who to?

- What do you think *should* happen? What values do you base your answer on? How do different ethical approaches come into play?

- What do you think *would* happen if this situation arose in your agency (or where you have been on placement)?

1   A social worker becomes engaged to a person who until two months ago was a user of the agency that employs the worker.

2   A social worker over-claims mileage allowance in order to fund a group for service users.

---

3 A social worker refuses to work with a same-sex couple because it contravenes his/her religious beliefs.

4 A social worker invites a service user to pray with him/her.

5 A social worker has many visible piercings and wears 'goth' style clothes and jewellery to work.

6 A social worker pays a service user to redecorate a room in the worker's house.

7 A social worker continues to visit a family occasionally as a friend, after the case has been transferred to another worker.

8 A social worker assists a severely disabled man to access sex sites on the internet.

9 A social worker is a member of a legal but extreme right-wing political party.

10 A social worker regularly asks colleagues in their office to lend them money.

11 A social worker accepts the offer of a glass of wine on a home visit to a family.

12 A social worker talks on Facebook about how often they go to clubs and get drunk.

Routine practice and decisions

Failings do not have to be as gross as physical abuse or theft, or even to involve going outside one's professional role, to have a damaging impact on people's lives. Official, authorised decisions and practice by staff who mean well can have harmful effects too, eating away at people's rights. The dangers of this are shown in the case of Steven Neary, a young man with learning disabilities and autism who was unlawfully deprived of his liberty for almost a full year in 2010. The judge concluded that everyone involved genuinely wanted the best for Steven, but in their desire to achieve this staff had failed to communicate honestly with his father. Furthermore, they had misused the deprivation of liberty safeguards (DOLS). These are meant to protect people from arbitrary detention, but staff had used them to prevent Steven from going home. The safeguards are summarised in Box 13.4. The case is *London Borough of Hillingdon v Neary and others* [2011].

Box 13.4: Deprivation of liberty safeguards (DOLS)

Article 5 of the ECHR is the right to liberty, but it is a limited right. Certain categories of people may be deprived of their liberty, including persons of 'unsound mind', provided it is done lawfully – that is, in accordance with a court order or sentence, or a legally authorised process. Criminal law and mental health law provide the main frameworks for this. Further, a person is not deprived of their liberty if they have the capacity to consent to the proposed action, and do so. But what about a person who does not meet the criteria for deprivation of liberty under criminal or mental health law, and cannot give valid consent – for example, someone with a severe learning disability or dementia. What protections are there for them?

The Mental Capacity Act applies in such cases (see Box 7.1). Any decision must be in the person's best interests, and the least restrictive option possible. There are additional protections if it is considered necessary to deprive someone of their liberty. The DOLS scheme applies to adults (over 18) in care homes or hospitals. If a deprivation of liberty is considered necessary for young people or adults in other settings, who cannot consent and cannot be detained under the Mental Health Act 1983, application has to be made to court – for adults, to the Court of Protection, and for children to the Family Division of the High Court.

The DOLS scheme was introduced into the Mental Capacity Act 2005, by the Mental Health Act 2007, in response to the judgment of the European Court of Human Rights in the case of *HL v United Kingdom* [2004] (the 'Bournewood judgment'). It came into force in April 2009. There is a DOLS Code of Practice (MoJ, 2008a). For a useful summary see SCIE (2011), and for highly critical views of the scheme for being unclear, over-complex and ineffective, two reports from the Mental Health Alliance (Hargreaves 2010, 2011).

Deprivation of liberty must be distinguished from restraint and restriction of liberty. It is possible for a person to be restrained or restricted without this amounting to a deprivation. The concepts are on a continuum, and the key factors are the 'degree and intensity' (see MoJ, 2008a: paras 2.1–2.12). A deprivation of liberty is not defined by the presence of one factor alone, even detaining someone in a particular place. Various aspects of controlling their care and movement may come under it – for example, continuous supervision or limiting their contact with other people. Other aspects to consider include the frequency, duration and number of restrictions. The law is complex and case law is developing fast (there is a useful summary in the judgment in *Cheshire West and Chester Council v P* [2011]).

Under the DOLS scheme, whenever it becomes apparent that a person is deprived of their liberty, or may become so in the next 28 days, the care home or the hospital ('the managing authority'), must apply for authorisation to the relevant supervisory body (at the time of writing, the local authority for care homes and the primary care trust for hospitals). In an emergency the managing authority may authorise urgent detention for up to seven days.

The supervisory body has to commission a deprivation of liberty assessment. This has six components, including mental capacity (the person must lack capacity to consent to the plan), mental health (they must have a mental disorder under the MHA 1983) and best interests (is the deprivation in their best interests, is it necessary to prevent harm to them, and is it proportionate?). The six tests must be undertaken by at least two different assessors, and in particular the mental health assessor and the best interests assessor must be different people. Regulations specify the training that must be undertaken by mental health assessors and best interests assessors.

If all six tests are satisfied, the supervisory body must authorise deprivation of liberty. This should be for the shortest possible period, in keeping with the principles of proportionality and using the least restrictive option, but may be for up to a year.

Steven Neary usually lived with his father, Mr Mark Neary, with a package of support from Hillingdon that included regular respite care. At times his behaviour could be very challenging. In December 2009, things became difficult and by the end of the month Mr Neary was unwell and exhausted. Steven was due for his regular one night period of respite care on 30 December 2009. He went to that, and the next day Mr Neary agreed for Steven to have an extended stay, 'for a couple of weeks' at a support unit. Just a few days later, on 4 January 2010, the social worker and the staff at the support unit had a meeting (without Mr Neary) and decided that Steven ought to stay for longer. The social worker told Mr Neary, who objected to a long-term stay. As things progressed throughout January, Mr Neary eventually agreed to a further short-term extension, but by then Hillingdon had decided that Steven should not go home for much longer. It did not reveal this to Mr Neary (para. 54 of the judgment).

The care home applied for DOLS authorisation in April 2010, following an incident when Steven wandered out of the unit. This was approved for two months, and then approved again in June 2010. Throughout this period, Mr Neary was not given a full account of Hillingdon's point of view, and thought the plan was that Steven would be coming back to live with him. When he did learn of their position, in early July, he immediately asked for Steven to be returned home (para. 103). Hillingdon refused to provide a package of care to support this. In desperation, Mr Neary started a Facebook campaign group, and the matter got considerable coverage in the local and national media.

In August 2010 Hillingdon decided that it would have to apply to the Court of Protection for an order settling where Steven should live. They eventually made the court application in late October 2010, and the case was heard in late December. (Meanwhile, the DOLS authorisation had been renewed in September and November 2010.) The judge ended the authorisation and Steven went home, with support services from Hillingdon.

A hearing was held in May 2011 to review the lawfulness of what had happened in 2010, in particular regarding the deprivation of liberty. The judge held that Steven had been detained unlawfully from 5 January onwards, even though there had been 'agreements' and DOLS authorisations. He said that Hillingdon had 'acted as if it had the right to make decisions about Steven, and by a combination of turning a deaf ear and force majeure, it tried to wear down Mr Neary's resistance' (para. 27).

The judge was critical of the standards of the best interests assessments (para. 174). These should be the cornerstone of the protection that the DOLS process offers to people, but they had not been adequate. Even though they had recommended deprivation of liberty, Hillingdon (as the supervisory authority) ought to have scrutinised them more carefully. One of the causes of difficulty in this case was that responsibilities and lines of accountability were blurred, because Hillingdon provided community-based services and social work support for Steven and his family, it ran the support unit (so it was the managing authority), and it was the supervisory body.

For all the criticism of Hillingdon, the judge also noted that they had provided extremely high levels of support to Steven and his family in the past, and said he was satisfied that 'everybody concerned has genuinely wanted to do the right thing by Steven at all times, and that a lot of hard work has been done to achieve this. The problems arose from misjudgement, not lack of commitment' (para. 16).

The key elements of Steven's case, namely the differences of opinion between people who were genuinely committed to his best interests, and the failures of communication about this, are frequent features of cases where disputes about deprivation of liberty reach the courts (MoJ, 2008a: para. 2.24). It is disturbing to read about the way that staff withheld information from Mr Neary, and about the poor quality assessments, but the story is typical of many cases that go wrong. No-one meant things to be as bad as they now look, but individuals suppressed their own misgivings, allowing organisational priorities to prevail. This is reflected in the evidence of the social work team manager, quoted in the judgment. He admitted that:

> There were times when we seriously questioned what we were doing and whether it was appropriate . . . I had periods of feeling extremely sure and moments when I myself questioned whether what we were doing was appropriate. In the end we determined to go forward. I didn't follow through on my doubts. There was momentum by that stage.
>
> (*London Borough of Hillingdon v Neary and others* [2011], para. 141).

Preston-Shoot (2011) is highly critical of the way that organisational culture and policies can create a gap between what professional ethics say and what happens in practice, and between what the law says on paper and how it is implemented in practice. He emphasises how great harm can be done through acts of routine practice and the unthinking following of rules, speaking of 'conformity interacting with a dulling of conscience' (Preston-Shoot, 2011: 186). Steven Neary's case shows how one-track thinking can sometimes come to dominate in an organisation, preventing staff from seeing the alternatives and acting on them.

Resources

If the desire to do the right thing can sometimes lead workers to override people's rights, the pressures of resource shortages are another major factor that threatens both service users' rights and the moral integrity of individual practitioners. The courts do not normally get involved in arguments about how much money social care services should have, holding that this is a political question, not a judicial matter. However, they will insist that whatever the budget, the decisions are made properly (legally, fairly, rationally and proportionately, as discussed in Chapter 3). This leads the courts to criticise social care departments in some cases, but to uphold their decisions in others.

The case of Elaine McDonald, heard by the Supreme Court in 2011, is an example of the court upholding the local authority's decision, but the judgment raises many questions about the realities of government policy of greater user choice and control (*R (McDonald) v Royal Borough of Kensington and Chelsea* [2011]; see also the earlier Court of Appeal judgment, *R (McDonald) v Royal Borough of Kensington and Chelsea* [2010]). It highlights the challenges of meeting people's wishes and needs in the context of limited resources.

Ms McDonald was a 67-year-old woman who, in her earlier life, had been a leading dancer with the Scottish Ballet. In 1999 she suffered a stroke that left her with reduced strength and mobility. In 2006–7 she had a number of falls, leading to periods in hospital. Although Ms McDonald was not incontinent, she had a bladder condition that meant she had to urinate several times during the night. She needed help to do this safely.

The issue was how this help should be provided. Ms McDonald was appalled at the idea of using incontinence pads or absorbent sheets, regarding these as an affront to her dignity. She wanted a night carer to help her get to a commode. The local authority was not prepared to agree to this, but did agree to provide it on a short-term basis while Ms McDonald applied for separate funding. Whether that application was ever made, or with what result, was not clear (para. 46 of the judgment), but after nearly two years the authority decided to reduce the amount allocated for her care because they did not consider that she needed a full-time night carer.

The authority's argument had two aspects. The first was financial. The cost of providing a night-time carer seven nights a week was over £22,000 per year, on top of day-time care. This would have had to come out of the budget for all adult care service users. Local authorities may take resources into account when assessing and deciding how to meet needs, but may not withdraw services without a reassessment (the *Barry* case, referred to in Chapter 3). There was a dispute about whether the case had been properly reassessed, but the court judged that it had. It accepted the local authority's argument, by a majority of 4–1, that Ms McDonald's essential need was to urinate safely, not to get to the commode. (The judge who disagreed, Lady Hale, did so strongly. She considered that Ms McDonald's need was indeed to use the commode, and that this should have been met.) The second part of the local authority's argument was that the need to urinate safely could better be met by the provision of pads. They argued that these were safer (avoiding the need to transfer to the commode) and gave more privacy and independence. They argued that other people in similar situations have been unhappy about the idea of pads, but have preferred them once they have tried them (para. 11). That may be so, but the fact remains, it was not Ms McDonald's choice.

Ms McDonald's case raises very hard but well-known questions about the realities of service provision, limited resources, the role of the courts and social work's ethical claims. Clements (2011) is scathing about the decision (his article is about the earlier Court of Appeal judgment, but that ruling was upheld by the Supreme Court). He argues that forcing Ms McDonald (who was continent) to use incontinence pads was contrary to her dignity, inconsistent with the values of a civilised society and indicative of the way that the human rights of vulnerable and older people are all too easily overridden by resource arguments. Lady Hale, in her dissenting judgment, also makes these points (and see Hale, 2009).

What then for social work? The international code of ethics in social work asserts that social workers should ensure that resources are distributed fairly, according to need, and that they have a duty to challenge unjust policies and practices:

> Social workers have a duty to bring to the attention of their employers, policy makers, politicians and the general public situations where resources are inadequate or where distribution of resources, policies and practice are oppressive, unfair or harmful.
>
> (IFSW and IASSW, 2004: para. 4.2.4)

(The BASW code of ethics uses identical wording, but adds 'or illegal' at the end: BASW, 2012: section 2.2.4). The quotation shows the radical, campaigning and advocacy side of social work, a side that is often squeezed out in local authority social care departments in England, where the focus is on responding to immediate, individual need, assessing eligibility for services and rationing resources.

Social work is familiar with the tensions between a categorical approach to people's rights and choices, and a utilitarian one, balancing them against the well-being of others. Self-determination is a prized value for social work, but is not the final word. The dilemmas are reflected in the following quotation from the international code (again, closely echoed in the 2012 BASW code, section 2.1.2):

> Social workers should respect and promote people's right to make their own choices and decisions, irrespective of their values and life choices, provided this does not threaten the rights and legitimate interests of others.
>
> (IFSW and IASSW, 2004: para. 4.1.1)

It is a simple sentence that captures a minefield of practical, ethical and legal dilemmas.

Conclusion

The organisational context is crucial to how well social workers do their jobs. There are three main possibilities: supporting, undermining, and blaming. The ethos and practices of a healthy organisation will use and support individual responsibility to bring about positive improvements. There will be room for individuals to question the ways that things get done, challenge poor practice, speak about the pressures, work with colleagues for change. Less healthy organisations will undermine a sense of individual responsibility ('just follow the procedures', 'that's the way we always do it'), or may try to deflect responsibility on to individuals in a blaming way ('they made a poor decision', 'they didn't follow the guidance', 'they couldn't cope').

One of the great challenges for social workers is to keep a sense of personal responsibility in the context of organisational requirements and pressures, to stay ethically engaged and alert to dangers and opportunities. It is important that workers continually ask themselves what are their own ethical responsibilities, thinking about categorical duties (the Kantian approach), the likely consequences (utilitarianism), how to maintain personal integrity (good character) and how best to show care. They have to consider how the policies of their organisation, and their own practice, help service users to achieve a better quality of life and as much autonomy as possible.

The law can be used to challenge social workers about whether and how they are truly helping service users – effectively protecting them from harm and enabling them to have as much control over their own lives as possible. At times, these challenges can be very uncomfortable for social workers and their agencies. But law can also be a resource for social workers, to help them safeguard individuals, empower them, and challenge oppressive policies and practices. Social workers do have to deal with the practical limitations of risk and resources; but even so, good social work can help people to live more independent and fulfilling lives. The rhetoric of autonomy and choice must not become an excuse for withholding services or blaming people ('they really ought to manage for themselves'), but a legal and ethical imperative for supporting people properly.

Questions for reflection

- What do you think you would you have done if you had been Steven Neary's social worker? Is it different to what you *hope* you would have done? (There is often a gap between what people say they would do in situations like that, and what they actually do.) What are the reasons for your answers?

- What do you think you would you have done if you had been Elaine McDonald's social worker? What do you hope you would have done? Are your answers different if you imagine yourself as the service manager? What are your reasons?

- What do you think you would you have done if you had been working at Winterbourne View? What do you hope you would have done?

Useful websites and further reading

Public Concern at Work: www.pcaw.org.uk

Clinic for Boundaries Studies (formerly 'Witness'): www.professionalboundaries.org.uk/Home.aspx

Care Quality Commission (regulator and inspector for adult social care): www.cqc.org.uk

Ofsted (regulator and inspector for children's social care): www.ofsted.gov.uk

GSCC (2011b) *Professional Boundaries: Guidance for Social Workers.*

Allen (2009) 'My brilliant survival guide'. This is a marvellous article, by Clare Allen, about her social worker. The reason for recommending it here is that it shows how the worker's clear professional and personal boundaries did not limit the helping relationship, but promoted it. Do read it, to inspire yourself about being a social worker!

Bibliography

Allen, C. (2009) 'My brilliant survival guide', *Guardian Society*, 14 January. Online. Available HTTP: <http://www. guardian.co.uk/society/2009/jan/14/mental-health-clare-allan-social-worker> (accessed 25 February 2012).

Allen, G. (2011) *Early Intervention: The Next Steps*, London: DfE. Online. Available HTTP: <http://www.dwp. gov.uk/docs/early-intervention-next-steps.pdf> (accessed 25 February 2012).

An-Na'im, A. (1994) 'Cultural transformation and normative consensus on the best interests of the child', *International Journal of Law and the Family*, 8: 62-81.

An-Na'im, A. (2000) *Forced Marriage*, paper commissioned by the Honour Crimes Project, School of Oriental and African Studies, London: SOAS. Online. Available HTTP: <http://www.soas.ac.uk/honourcrimes/resources/ file55689.pdf> (accessed 25 February 2012).

Aristotle (350 BCE) *Nicomachean Ethics*. Translated by W. D. Ross (1908), Oxford: Clarendon Press. Online. Available HTTP: <http://classics.mit.edu/Aristotle/nicomachaen.html> (accessed 25 February 2012).

Ayre, P. and Preston-Shoot, M. (eds) (2010) *Children's Services at the Crossroads: A Critical Evaluation of Contemporary Policy for Practice*, Lyme Regis: Russell House Publishing.

Baggini, J. (2011) 'England riots: are harsh sentences for offenders justified?', *The Guardian*, (G2 supplement, 18 August). Online. Available HTTP: <http://www.guardian.co.uk/uk/2011/aug/17/england-riots-harsh-sentences-justified> (accessed 25 February 2012).

Bailey, R. and Brake, M. (eds) (1975) *Radical Social Work*, London: Edward Arnold.

Bailey-Harris R. and Harris, M. (2002) 'Local authorities and child protection - the mosaic of accountability', *Child and Family Law Quarterly*, 14(2): 117-36.

Ball, C., Harris, R., Roberts, G. and Vernon, S. (1988) *The Law Report: Teaching and Assessment of Law in Social Work Education*, London: CCETSW.

Banks, S. (1999) 'The social professions and social policy: proactive or reactive?', *European Journal of Social Work*, 2: 327-39.

Banks, S. (2004) *Ethics, Accountability and the Social Professions*, Basingstoke: Palgrave Macmillan.

Banks, S. (2010) 'Integrity in professional life: issues of conduct, commitment and capacity', *British Journal of Social Work*, 40: 2168-84.

Banks, S. (2012) *Ethics and Values in Social Work*, 4th edn, Basingstoke: Palgrave Macmillan/BASW.

Banks, S. and Gallagher, A. (2009) *Ethics in Professional Life*, Basingstoke: Palgrave Macmillan.

Barber, P., Brown, R. and Martin, D. (2012) *Mental Health Law in England and Wales*, 2nd edn, London: Sage/ Learning Matters.

Barkham, P. (2008) 'Hannah's choice', *The Guardian, G2* section, 12 November. Online. Available HTTP: <http://www.guardian.co.uk/society/2008/nov/12/health-child-protection> (accessed 25 February 2012).

Barnard, A., Horner, N. and Wild, J. (eds) (2008) *The Value Base of Social Work and Social Care*, Maidenhead: Open University Press.

BASW (British Association of Social Workers) (2002) *Code of Ethics*, Birmingham: BASW. Online. Available HTTP: <http://www.basw.co.uk/about/code-of-ethics/> (accessed 25 February 2012).

BASW (2012) *Code of Ethics in Social Work: Statement of Principles*, Birmingham: BASW. Online. Available HTTP: <http://www.basw.co.uk/codeofethics/> (accessed 25 February 2012).

Bauman, Z. (1993) *Postmodern Ethics*, Oxford; Blackwell.

Bazalgette, L. and Bradley, W. (2010) *Commission on Assisted Dying Briefing Paper: Key Research Themes*, London: Demos. Online. Available HTTP: <http://www.commissiononassisteddying.co.uk/wp-content/uploads/2010/11/Demos-Briefing-Paper-The-Commission-on-Assisted-Dying-Key-Research-Themes.pdf> (accessed 25 February 2012).

Bebbington, A. and Miles, J. (1989) 'The background of children who enter local authority care', *British Journal of Social Work*, 19: 349-78.

Beckett, C. (2001) 'Children who wait for courts: legal delays in care proceedings', *British Journal of Social Work*, 31: 317-23.

Beckett, C. and Maynard, A. (2005) *Values and Ethics in Social Work: An Introduction*, London: Sage

Bentham, J. (1780) *Introduction to the Principles of Morals and Legislation*. Online. Available HTTP: <http://www.utilitarianism.com> (accessed 25 February 2012).

Beresford, P., Adshead, L. and Croft, S. (2007) *Palliative Care, Social Work and Service Users: Making Life Possible*, London: Jessica Kingsley.

Berger, P. and Luckmann, T. (1967) *The Social Construction of Reality*, London: Penguin.

BIHR (British Institute for Human Rights) (2008) *The Human Rights Act: Changing Lives*, 2nd edn, London: BIHR. Online. Available HTTP: <http://www.bihr.org.uk/documents/policy/changing-lives-second-edition> (accessed 25 February 2012).

Bingham, T. (2010) *The Rule of Law*, London: Allen Lane.

Blackburn, C., Spencer, N. and Read, J. (2010) 'Prevalence of childhood disability and the characteristics and circumstances of disabled children in the UK: secondary analysis of the Family Resources Survey', *BMC Paediatrics*, 10: 21-32.

Blofield, J. (2004) *Independent Inquiry into the Death of David Bennett*, Cambridge: Norfolk, Suffolk and Cambridgeshire Strategic Health Authority. Online. Available HTTP: <https://www.eoe.nhs.uk/page.php?page_id=179> (accessed 25 February 2012).

Blom-Cooper, L. and Drewry, G. (eds) (1976) *Law and Morality*, London: Duckworth.

Bogg, D. (2010) *Values and Ethics in Mental Health Practice*, Exeter: Learning Matters.

Booth, M. (1996) *Avoiding Delay in Children Act Cases*, London: LCD.

Bowers, J., Fodder, M., Lewis, J. and Mitchell, J. (2007) *Whistleblowing: Law and Practice*, 2nd edn, Oxford: Oxford University press.

Bowers, M. and Dubicka, B. (2009) 'Legal dilemmas for clinicians involved in the care and treatment of children and young people with mental disorder', *Child: Care, Health and Development*, 36: 592-6.

Brammer, A. (2010) *Social Work Law*, 3rd edn, Harlow: Pearson.

Brandon, M., Belderson, P., Warren, C., Howe, D., Gardner, R., Dodsworth, J. and Black, J. (2008) *Analysing Child Deaths and Serious Injury Through Abuse and Neglect: What Can We Learn? A Biennial Analysis of Serious Case Reviews 2003-2005*, London: DCSF. Online. Available HTTP: <http://webarchive.nationalarchives.gov.uk/20080305115902/dcsf.gov.uk/research/data/uploadfiles/dcsf-rr023.pdf> (accessed 25 February 2012).

Brandon, M., Bailey, S., Belderson, P., Gardner, R., Sidebotham, P., Dodsworth, J., Warren, C. and Black, J. (2009) *Understanding Serious Case Reviews and their Impact: A Biennial Analysis of Serious Case Reviews*

2005-07, DCSF Research Report 129, London: DCSF. Online. Available HTTP: <https://www.education.gov.uk/publications/eOrderingDownload/DCSF-RR129(R).pdf> (accessed 25 February 2012).

Brandon, M., Bailey, S. and Belderson, P. (2010) *Building on the Learning from Serious Case Reviews: A Two-Year Analysis of Child Protection Database Notifications 2007-2009*, London: DfE. Online. Available HTTP: <https://www.education.gov.uk/publications/RSG/AllPublications/Page1/DFE-RR040> (accessed 25 February 2012).

Braye, S. and Preston-Shoot, M. (1990) 'On teaching and applying the law in social work practice: it is not that simple', *British Journal of Social Work*, 20: 333-53.

Braye, S. and Preston-Shoot, M. (2006) 'The role of law in welfare reform: critical perspectives on the relationship between law and social work practice', *International Journal of Social Welfare*, 15: 19-26.

Braye, S. and Preston-Shoot, M. (2010) *Practising Social Work Law*, 3rd edn, Basingstoke: Palgrave Macmillan/BASW.

Brayne, H. and Carr, H. (2010) *Law for Social Workers*, 11th edn, Oxford: OUP.

Brent, London Borough of (1985) *A Child in Trust: The Report of the Panel of Inquiry Investigating the Circumstances Surrounding the Death of Jasmine Beckford*, London: London Borough of Brent.

Brophy, J. (2006) *Research Review: Child Care Proceedings under the Children Act 1989*, DCA Research Series 5/06, London: MoJ. Online. Available HTTP: <http://webarchive.nationalarchives.gov.uk/20090117123427/http://www.dca.gov.uk/research/2006/05_2006.pdf> (accessed 25 February 2012).

Brown, R. and Barber, P. (2008) *The Social Worker's Guide to the Mental Capacity Act 2005*, Exeter: Learning Matters.

Buckley, H. (2005) 'Neglect: no monopoly on expertise' in Taylor, J. and Daniel, B. (eds) *Child Neglect: Practice Issues for Health and Social Care*, London: Jessica Kingsley Publishers.

Burgess, A. (1962) *A Clockwork Orange*, London: Heinemann.

CAADA (Co-ordinated Action Against Domestic Abuse) (2007) *Disclosure of Information During and After MARAC Meetings: Frequently Asked Questions*. Online. Available HTTP: <http://www.caada.org.uk/marac/Resources_for_people_who_refer_to_MARAC.html> (accessed 25 February 2012).

CAD (Commission on Assisted Dying) (2012) *Report of the Commission on Assisted Dying*, London: Demos. Online. Available HTTP: <http://www.demos.co.uk/publications/thecommissiononassisteddying> (accessed 25 February 2012).

Cameron, D. (2011) *The Fightback after the Riots*, speech given on 15 August, Oxfordshire. Online. Available HTTP: <http://www.number10.gov.uk/news/pms-speech-on-the-fightback-after-the-riots/> (accessed 25 February 2012).

Campbell, B. (1988) *Unofficial Secrets. Child Sexual Abuse: The Cleveland Case*, London: Virago.

Campbell, J. (2008) 'It's my life - it's my decision? Assisted dying versus assisted living' in Clements, L. and Read, J. (eds) *Disabled People and the Right to Life: The Protection and Violation of Disabled People's Most Basic Human Rights*, Abingdon: Routledge.

Campbell, J. and Davidson, G. (2009) 'Coercion in the community: a situated approach to the examination of ethical challenges for mental health social workers', *Ethics and Social Welfare*, 3(3): 249-63.

Carr, S. (2010) *Enabling Risk, Ensuring Safety: Self-Directed Support and Personal Budgets*, SCIE Report 36, London: SCIE. Online. Available HTTP: <http://www.scie.org.uk/publications/reports/report36/> (accessed 25 February 2012).

Cassidy, D. and Davey, S. (2011) *Family Justice Children's Proceedings - Review of Public and Private Law Case Files in England and Wales*, Ministry of Justice Research Summary 5/11, London: MoJ. Online. Available HTTP: <http://www.justice.gov.uk/publications/research-and-analysis/moj/family-justice-children.htm> (accessed 25 February 2012).

Children's Commissioner for England (2010) *The Views of Children and Young People Regarding Media Access to Family Courts*, London: Children's Commissioner for England. Online. Available HTTP: <http://www.childrenscommissioner.gov.uk/content/publications/content_397> (accessed 25 February 2012).

Children's Society (2011) *4 in every 10 Disabled Children Living in Poverty*. London: Children's Society. Online. Available HTTP: <http://www.childrenssociety.org.uk/sites/default/files/tcs/4_in_10_reportfinal.pdf> (accessed 25 February 2012).

Christie, N. (1977) 'Conflicts as property', *British Journal of Criminology*, 17(1): 1-15.

Clark, C. (2000) *Social Work Ethics: Politics, Principles and Practice*, London: Macmillan.

Clark, C. (2006a) 'Moral character in social work', *British Journal of Social Work*, 36: 75-89.

Clark, C. (2006b) 'Against confidentiality: privacy, safety and the public good in professional communications', *Journal of Social Work*, 6: 117-36.

Clark, C. and McGhee, J. (eds) (2008) *Private and Confidential: Handling Personal Information in the Social and Health Services*, Bristol: Policy Press.

Clements, L. (2011) 'Social care law developments: a sideways look at personalisation and tightening eligibility criteria', *Elder Law*, 1: 47-52. Pre-publication draft online. Available HTTP: <http://www.lukeclements.co.uk/downloads/ElderLawArticleJan2011.pdf> (accessed 25 February 2012).

Clements, L. and Read, J. (eds) (2008) *Disabled People and the Right to Life: The Protection and Violation of Disabled People's Most Basic Human Rights*, Abingdon: Routledge.

Clements, L. and Thompson, P. (2011) *Community Care and the Law*, 5th edn, London: Legal Action Group.

Commission on Funding of Care and Support (2011) *Fairer Care Funding* ('The Dilnot Report'), London: Commission on Funding of Care and Support. Online. Available HTTP: <http://www.dilnotcommission.dh.gov.uk/> (accessed 25 February 2012).

CQC (Care Quality Commission) (2011) *CQC Review of Castlebeck Group Services*, London: CQC. Online. Available HTTP: <http://www.cqc.org.uk/public/our-action-winterbourne-view#cr> (accessed 25 February 2012).

Craig, C., Burchardt, T. and Gordon, D. (eds) (2008) *Social Justice and Public Policy: Seeking Fairness in Diverse Societies*, Bristol: Policy Press.

CSPL (Committee on Standards in Public Life) (2005) *Getting the Balance Right: Implementing Standards of Conduct in Public Life*, Tenth Report of the Committee. London: CSPL. Online. Available HTTP: <http://www.public-standards.gov.uk/OurWork/Tenth_Report.html> (accessed 25 February 2012).

Cunneen, C. and Hoyle, C. (2010) *Debating Restorative Justice*, Oxford: Hart Publishing.

Davies, C. and Ward, H. (2011) *Safeguarding Children Across Services: Messages from Research*, London: Jessica Kingsley Publishers. Online. Available HTTP: <https://www.education.gov.uk/publications/eOrderingDownload/DFE-RR164.pdf> (accessed 25 February 2012).

Davis, L. (2009) *The Social Worker's Guide to Children and Families Law*, London: Jessica Kingsley Publishers.

Day, E. (2009) 'Baby RB: heartbreak in Court 50 as life of a one-year-old hangs in the balance', *The Observer*, 8 November. Online. Available HTTP: <http://www.guardian.co.uk/society/2009/nov/08/baby-rb-court-case> (accessed 25 February 2012).

DCA (Department for Constitutional Affairs) (2006a) *Human Rights, Human Lives: A Handbook for Public Authorities*, London: DCA. Online. Available HTTP: <http://webarchive.nationalarchives.gov.uk/+/http://www.justice.gov.uk/docs/hr-handbook-public-authorities.pdf> (accessed 25 February 2012).

DCA (2006b) *Review of the Implementation of the Human Rights Act*, London: DCA. Online. Available HTTP: <http://webarchive.nationalarchives.gov.uk/+/http://www.justice.gov.uk/guidance/docs/full_review.pdf> (accessed 25 February 2012).

DCA (2006c) *Confidence and Confidentiality: Improving Transparency and Privacy in Family Courts*, Cm 6886, Norwich: TSO. Online. Available HTTP: <http://webarchive.nationalarchives.gov.uk/+/http://www.dca.gov.uk/consult/courttransparencey1106/cp1106.htm> (accessed 25 February 2012).

DCA (2007a) *Mental Capacity Act 2005 Code of Practice*, London: TSO. Online. Available HTTP: <http://webarchive.nationalarchives.gov.uk/+/http://www.dca.gov.uk/legal-policy/mental-capacity/mca-cp.pdf> (accessed 25 February 2012).

DCA (2007b) *Confidence and Confidentiality: Improving Transparency and Privacy in Family Courts - Response to Consultation*, London: DCA. Online. Available HTTP: <http://webarchive.nationalarchives.gov.uk/+/http://www.dca.gov.uk/consult/courttransparencey1106/cp1106.htm> (accessed 25 February 2012).

DCSF (Department for Children, Schools and Families) and Cafcass (2008) *Parenting Plans: Putting Your Children First. A Guide for Separating Parents*, London: DCSF and Cafcass. Online. Available HTTP: <http://www.cafcass.gov.uk/PDF/FINAL%20web%20version%20251108.pdf> (accessed 25 February 2012).

DfE (Department for Education) (2011a) *A Child-Centred System: The Government's Response to the Munro Review of Child Protection*, London: DfE. Online. Available HTTP: <http://www.education.gov.uk/munroreview/downloads/GovernmentResponsetoMunro.pdf> (accessed 25 February 2012).

DfE (2011b) *Characteristics of Children in Need in England, Final*, OSR26/2011, London: DfE. Online. Available HTTP: <http://media.education.gov.uk/assets/files/pdf/o/main%20text%20osr262011.pdf> (accessed 25 February 2012).

DfES (Department for Education and Skills), DCA and Welsh Assembly Government (2006) *Review of the Child Care Proceedings System in England and Wales*, London: DfES. Online. Available HTTP: <http://webarchive.nationalarchives.gov.uk/+/http://www.dca.gov.uk/publications/reports_reviews/childcare_ps.pdf> (accessed 25 February 2012).

DH (Department of Health) (2003) *Fair Access to Care Services: Guidance on Eligibility Criteria for Adult Social Care*, LAC (2003)12, London: DH. Online. Available HTTP: <http://www.dh.gov.uk/en/Publicationsandstatistics/Publications/PublicationsPolicyAndGuidance/DH_4009653> (accessed 25 February 2012).

DH (2004) *Best Practice Guidance for Doctors and other Health Professionals on the Provision of Advice and Treatment to Young People under 16 on Contraception, Sexual and Reproductive Health*, London: DH. Online. Available HTTP: <http://www.dh.gov.uk/en/Publicationsandstatistics/Publications/PublicationsPolicyAndGuidance/DH_4086960> (accessed 25 February 2012).

DH (2005) *Delivering Race Equality in Mental Health Care: An Action Plan for Reform Inside and Outside Services and the Government's Response to the Independent Inquiry into the Death of David Bennett*, London: DH. Online. Available HTTP: <http://www.dh.gov.uk/en/Publicationsandstatistics/Publications/PublicationsPolicyAndGuidance/DH_4100773> (accessed 25 February 2012).

DH (2007) *Independence, Choice and Risk: A Guide to Best Practice in Supported Decision-Making*, London: DH. Online. Available HTTP: <http://www.dh.gov.uk/en/Publicationsandstatistics/Publications/PublicationsPolicyAndGuidance/DH_074773> (accessed 25 February 2012).

DH (2008a) *Putting People First: Transforming Adult Social Care: The Whole Story*, London: DH. Online. Available HTTP: <http://www.dh.gov.uk/en/Publicationsandstatistics/Publications/PublicationsPolicyAndGuidance/DH_089665> (accessed 25 February 2012).

DH (2008b) *Code of Practice: Mental Health Act 1983*, Norwich: TSO. Online. Available HTTP: <http://www.dh.gov.uk/en/Publicationsandstatistics/Publications/PublicationsPolicyAndGuidance/DH_084597> (accessed 25 February 2012).

DH (2009) *Safeguarding Adults: Report on the Consultation on the Review of 'No Secrets'*, London: DH. Online. Available HTTP: <http://www.dh.gov.uk/prod_consum_dh/groups/dh_digitalassets/documents/digitalasset/dh_102981.pdf> (accessed 25 February 2012).

DH (2010a) *Practical Approaches to Safeguarding and Personalisation*, London: DH. Online. Available HTTP: <http://www.dh.gov.uk/prod_consum_dh/groups/dh_digitalassets/@dh/@en/@ps/documents/digitalasset/dh_121671.pdf> (accessed 25 February 2012).

DH (2010b) *Prioritising Need in the Context of Putting People First: A Whole System Approach to Eligibility for Social Care: Guidance on Eligibility Criteria for Social Care*, London: DH. Online. Available HTTP: <http://www.dh.gov.uk/en/Publicationsandstatistics/Publications/PublicationsPolicyAndGuidance/DH_113154> (accessed 25 February 2012).

DH, Department of Education and Employment and Home Office (2000) *Framework for the Assessment of Children in Need and their Families*, London: TSO. Online. Available HTTP: <http://www.dh.gov.uk/en/Publicationsand statistics/Publications/PublicationsPolicyAndGuidance/DH_4008144> (accessed 25 February 2012).

DHSS (Department of Health and Social Security) (1988) *Report of the Inquiry into Child Abuse in Cleveland 1987*, Cm 412, London: HMSO.

Dickens, J. (2004) 'Risks and responsibilities: the role of the local authority lawyer in child care cases', *Child and Family Law Quarterly*, 16(1): 17-30.

Dickens, J. (2005) 'Being "the epitome of reason": the challenges for lawyers and social workers in child care proceedings', *International Journal of Law, Policy and the Family*, 19(1): 1-29.

Dickens, J. (2006) 'Social work, law, money and trust: paying for lawyers in child protection work', *Journal of Social Welfare and Family Law*, 28(3-4): 283-95.

Dickens, J. (2007) 'Child neglect and the law: catapults, thresholds and delay', *Child Abuse Review*, 16: 77-92.

Dickens, J. (2011) 'Social work in England at a watershed - as always: from the Seebohm report to the Social Work Task Force', *British Journal of Social Work*, 41: 22-39.

Dickens, J. (2012) 'The definition of social work in the United Kingdom, 2000-2010', *International Journal of Social Welfare*, 21: 34-43.

Dignity in Dying (2006) *Dignity in Dying: The Report*, London: Dignity in Dying. Online. Available HTTP: <http://www.dignityindying.org.uk/includes/spaw2/uploads/files/Dignity%20in%20Dying%20Report.pdf> (accessed 25 February 2012).

Dingwall, R., Eekelaar, J. and Murray, T. (1983) *The Protection of Children: State Intervention and Family Life*, Oxford: Basil Blackwell (2nd edn 1995, Aldershot: Avebury).

Doel, M., Allmark, P., Conway, P., Cowburn, M., Flynn, M., Nelson, P. and Tod, A. (2009) *Professional Boundaries: Research Report*. Report to the General Social Care Council. Sheffield: Sheffield Hallam University. Online. Available HTTP: <http://www.gscc.org.uk/cmsFiles/Publications/GSCC_Professional_Boundaries_Research_Report_2009.pdf> (accessed 25 February 2012).

Doel, M., Allmark, P., Conway, P., Cowburn, M., Flynn, M., Nelson, P. and Tod, A. (2010) 'Professional boundaries: crossing the line or entering the shadows?', *British Journal of Social Work*, 40: 1866-89.

Dominelli, l. (2002) *Anti-Oppressive Social Work Theory and Practice*, Basingstoke: Palgrave Macmillan.

Dominelli, L. (2009) *Introducing Social Work*, Cambridge: Polity.

Dorling, D. (2010) *Injustice: Why Social Inequality Persists*, Bristol: Policy Press.

Douglas, M. (1992) 'The retreat from Gillick', *Modern Law Review*, 55(4): 569-76.

DPP (Director of Public Prosecutions) (2010) *Policy for Prosecutors in Respect of Cases of Encouraging or Assisting Suicide*, London: Crown Prosecution Service. Online. Available HTTP: <http://www.cps.gov.uk/publications/prosecution/assisted_suicide_policy.html> (accessed 25 February 2012).

Durkheim, E. (1895) *The Rules of Sociological Method*. Translated by W. D. Halls (1982), New York: The Free Press.

Edemariam, A. (2009) 'A double agent, that's what I was', interview with Margaret Haywood, *The Guardian*, 14 November. Online. Available HTTP: <http://www.guardian.co.uk/society/2009/nov/14/margaret-haywood-double-agent> (accessed 25 February 2012).

Eekelaar, J. and Dingwall, R. (1990) *The Reform of Child Care Law*, London: Routledge.

Eekelaar, J., Maclean, M. and Beinhart, S. (2000) *Family Lawyers: The Divorce Work of Solicitors*, Oxford: Hart Publishing.

EHRC (Equality and Human Rights Commission) (2008) *Ours to Own: Understanding Human Rights*, London: EHRC. Online. Available HTTP: <http://www.equalityhumanrights.com/human-rights/human-rights-practical-guidance/guidance-from-the-commission/> (accessed 25 February 2012).

EHRC (2009) *Human Rights Inquiry*, London: EHRC. Online. Available HTTP: <http://www.equalityhumanrights.com/human-rights/our-human-rights-inquiry/> (accessed 25 February 2012).

EHRC (2010) *How Fair is Britain? First Triennial Review*, London: EHRC. Online. Available HTTP: <http://www.equalityhumanrights.com/key-projects/how-fair-is-britain/> (accessed 25 February 2012).

EHRC (2011a) *Hidden in Plain Sight: Inquiry into Disability-Related Harassment*, London: EHRC. Online. Available HTTP: <http://www.equalityhumanrights.com/legal-and-policy/inquiries-and-assessments/inquiry-into-disability-related-harassment/> (accessed 25 February 2012).

EHRC (2011b) *Close to Home: An Inquiry into Older People and Human Rights in Home Care*, London: EHRC. Online. Available HTTP: <http://www.equalityhumanrights.com/legal-and-policy/inquiries-and-assessments/inquiry-into-home-care-of-older-people/> (accessed 25 February 2012).

Equalities Review (2007) *Fairness and Freedom: The Final Report of the Equalities Review*, London: Equalities Review. Online. Available HTTP: <http://www.communities.gov.uk/publications/corporate/fairnessfreedom> (accessed 25 February 2012).

Fairbairn, C. and Gheera, M. (2009) *Transparency in the Family Courts*, Parliamentary Briefing Paper, SN/HA/4844, London: House of Commons Library. Online. Available HTTP: <http://www.parliament.uk/briefing-papers/SN04844> (accessed 25 February 2012).

Farmer, E. and Lutman, E. (2010) *Case Management and Outcomes for Neglected Children Returned to their Parents: A Five Year Follow-Up Study*, DCSF Research Brief RB214, London: DfE. Online. Available HTTP: <https://www.education.gov.uk/publications/standard/publicationdetail/page1/DCSF-RB214> (accessed 25 February 2012).

Featherstone, B. (2010) 'Ethic of care' in Gray, M. and Webb, S. *Ethics and Value Perspectives in Social Work*, Basingstoke: Palgrave Macmillan.

Ferguson, H. (2011) *Child Protection Practice*, Basingstoke: Palgrave Macmillan.

Ferguson, I. (2007) 'Increasing user choice or privatizing risk? The antinomies of personalization', *British Journal of Social Work*, 37: 387–403.

Ferguson, I. and Woodward, R. (2009) *Radical Social Work in Practice*, Bristol: Policy Press.

Field, F. (2010) *The Foundation Years: Preventing Poor Children Becoming Poor Adults*, London: HM Government. Online. Available HTTP: <http://webarchive.nationalarchives.gov.uk/20110120090128/http:/povertyreview.independent.gov.uk> (accessed 25 February 2012).

FJR (Family Justice Review) (2011a) *Interim Report*, London: MoJ. Online. Available HTTP: <http://www.justice.gov.uk/about/moj/independent-reviews/family-justice-review/> (accessed 25 February 2012).

FJR (2011b) *Final Report*, London: MoJ. Online. Available HTTP: <http://www.justice.gov.uk/about/moj/independent-reviews/family-justice-review/> (accessed 25 February 2012).

FMU (Forced Marriage Unit) (2011) *Dealing with Forced Marriages*, e-learning module. Online. Available HTTP: <http://www.fco.gov.uk/en/travel-and-living-abroad/when-things-go-wrong/forced-marriage/info-for-professionals> (accessed 25 February 2012).

Fortin, J. (2006) 'Accommodating children's rights in a post Human Rights Act era', *Modern Law Review*, 69(3): 299–326.

Fortin, J. (2009) *Children's Rights and the Developing Law*, 3rd edn, Cambridge: Cambridge University Press.

Foucault, M. (1977) *Discipline and Punish: The Birth of the Prison* (first published in French, 1975), Harmondsworth: Penguin.

Fyson, R. and Kitson, D. (2010) 'Human rights and social wrongs: issues in safeguarding adults with learning disabilities', *Practice*, 22(5): 309–20.

Galanter, M. (1974) 'Why the "haves" come out ahead: speculations on the limits of legal change', *Law and Society*, 9: 95–160.

Ghate, D. and Hazel, N. (2002) *Parenting in Poor Environments: Stress, Support and Coping*, London: Jessica Kingsley. Summary published by Policy Research Bureau, Online. Available HTTP: <http://www.prb.org.uk/publications/P150%20Parenting%20Summary.pdf> (accessed 25 February 2012).

Giddens, A. (1984). *The Constitution of Society: Outline of the Theory of Structuration*, Cambridge: Polity Press.

Gill, A. (2011) *Exploring the Viability of Creating a Specific Offence of Forced Marriage in England and Wales: Report on Findings*, London: University of Roehampton. Online. Available HTTP: <http://www.avaproject.org.uk/media/68857/forced-marriage-legislation-survey_report-of-findings_gill_13july_final.pdf> (accessed 25 February 2012).

Gilligan, C. (1982) *In a Different Voice*, Cambridge, Mass.: Harvard University Press.

GMC (General Medical Council) (2010) *Treatment and Care Towards the End of Life: Good Practice in Decision-Making*, London: GMC. Online. Available HTTP: <http://www.gmc-uk.org/guidance/ethical_guidance/end_of_life_care.asp> (accessed 25 February 2012).

Gray, M. (2010) 'Moral sources and emergent ethical theories in social work', *British Journal of Social Work*, 40: 1794-811.

Gray, M. and Webb, S. (eds) (2010) *Ethics and Value Perspectives in Social Work*, Basingstoke: Palgrave Macmillan.

Greene, A. and Kantambu Latting, J. (2004) 'Whistle-blowing as a form of advocacy: guidelines for the practitioner and organization', *Social Work*, 49(2): 219-30.

Greenwich, London Borough of (1987) *A Child in Trust: Protection of Children in a Responsible Society. Report of the Commission of Inquiry into the Circumstances Surrounding the Death of Kimberley Carlile*, London: London Borough of Greenwich.

Gregory, M. (2010) 'Reflection and resistance: probation practice and the ethic of care', *British Journal of Social Work*, 40: 2274-90.

GSCC (General Social Care Council) (2002a) *Code of Practice for Social Care Workers and Code of Practice for Social Care Employers*, London: GSCC. Online. Available HTTP: <http://www.gscc.org.uk/codes/> (accessed 25 February 2012).

GSCC (2002b) *Accreditation of Universities to Award Degrees in Social Work*, London: GSCC. Online. Available HTTP: <http://www.gscc.org.uk/cmsFiles/Education%20and%20Training/Accreditation%20of%20universities%20to%20grant%20degrees%20in%20social%20work.pdf> (accessed 25 February 2012).

GSCC (2008) *Raising Standards: Social Work Conduct in England 2003-08*, London: GSCC. Online. Available HTTP: <http://www.gscc.org.uk/page/193/Conduct+publications.htm> (accessed 25 February 2012).

GSCC (2010a) *Notice of Decision of the Conduct Committee: Ms Gillie Christou*, London: CSCC. Available HTTP: <http://www.gscc.org.uk/page/246/2010-11.html#May> (accessed 25 February 2012).

GSCC (2010b) *Notice of Decision of the Conduct Committee: Ms Maria Ward*, London: GSCC. Available HTTP: <http://www.gscc.org.uk/page/246/2010-11.html#May> (accessed 25 February 2012).

GSCC (2010c) *Social Work in Mental Health Services: Specialist Standards and Requirements for Post-Qualifying Social Work Education and Training*, revised edn, London: GSCC. Online. Available HTTP: <http://www.gscc.org.uk/cmsFiles/Education%20and%20Training/PQ%20documents/Social%20work%20in%20mental%20health%20services%20revised%202010.pdf> (accessed 25 February 2012).

GSCC (2011a) 'GSCC issues guidance to help social workers manage professional boundaries', *GSCC Press Release*, 21 November. Online. Available HTTP: <http://www.gscc.org.uk/news/40/Professional-Boundaries-guidance-launch.html> (accessed 25 February 2012).

GSCC (2011b) *Professional Boundaries: Guidance for Social Workers*, London: GSCC. Online. Available HTTP: <http://www.gscc.org.uk/page/326/Professional+Boundaries.html> (accessed 25 February 2012).

Hale, B. (2009) 'Dignity', *Journal of Social Welfare and Family Law*, 31(2): 101-8.

Hargreaves, R. (2010) *Deprivation of Liberty Safeguards: An Initial Review of Implementation*, London: Mental Health Alliance. Online. Available HTTP: <http://www.mentalhealthalliance.org.uk/resources/DoLS_report_July2010.pdf> (accessed 25 February 2012).

Hargreaves, R. (2011) *The Deprivation of Liberty Safeguards (DoLS): Pre-Publication Draft v2*, London: Mental Health Alliance. Online. Available HTTP: <http://www.mentalhealthalliance.org.uk/news/DoLS_study.html> (accessed 25 February 2012).

Haringey LSCB (Local Safeguarding Children Board) (2008) *Serious Case Review 'Child A'*, London: DfE. Online. Available HTTP: <http://education.gov.uk/inthenews/inthenews/a0065565/peter-connelly-serious-case-review-reports-published> (accessed 25 February 2012).

Haringey LSCB (2009) *Serious Case Review 'Child A': Second Serious Case Review Overview Report Relating to Peter Connelly*, London: DfE. Online. Available HTTP: <http://education.gov.uk/inthenews/inthenews/a0065565/peter-connelly-serious-case-review-reports-published> (accessed 25 February 2012).

Healy, K. (2007) 'Universalism and cultural relativism in social work ethics' *International Social Work*, 50(1): 11–26.

Held, V. (2006) *The Ethics of Care: Personal, Political and Global*, Oxford: OUP.

Hill, A. (2010) *Working in Statutory Contexts*, Cambridge: Polity.

HM Government (2008a) *The Right to Choose: Multi-Agency Statutory Guidance for Dealing with Forced Marriage*, London: Forced Marriage Unit Online. Available HTTP: <http://www.fco.gov.uk/resources/en/pdf/3849543/forced-marriage-right-to-choose> (accessed 25 February 2012).

HM Government (2008b) *Information Sharing: Guidance for Practitioners and Managers*, London: DCSF. Online. Available HTTP: <http://www.education.gov.uk/childrenandyoungpeople/strategy/integratedworking/a0072915/information-sharing> (accessed 25 February 2012).

HM Government (2009a) *Multi-Agency Practice Guidelines: Handing Cases of Forced Marriage*, London: Forced Marriage Unit Online. Available HTTP: <http://www.fco.gov.uk/resources/en/pdf/3849543/forced-marriage-guidelines09.pdf> (accessed 25 February 2012).

HM Government (2009b) *Information Sharing: Further Guidance on Legal Issues*, London: DCSF Online. Available HTTP: <http://www.education.gov.uk/childrenandyoungpeople/strategy/integratedworking/a0072915/information-sharing> (accessed 25 February 2012).

HM Government (2010a) *The Equality Strategy: Building a Fairer Britain*, Online. Available HTTP: <http://www.homeoffice.gov.uk/publications/equalities/equality-strategy-publications/equality-strategy/> (accessed 25 February 2012).

HM Government (2010b) *The Children Act 1989 Guidance and Regulations, Volume 2: Care Planning, Placement and Case Review*, Nottingham: DCSF. Online. Available HTTP: <http://www.education.gov.uk/childrenandyoungpeople/families/childrenincare/a0065502/care-planning-for-looked-after-children-and-care-leavers> (accessed 25 February 2012).

HM Government (2010c) *Working Together to Safeguard Children*, Nottingham: DCSF. Online. Available HTTP: <https://www.education.gov.uk/publications/standard/publicationdetail/page1/DCSF-00305-2010> (accessed 25 February 2012).

HM Government (2010d) *Forced Marriage and Learning Disabilities: Multi-Agency Practice Guidance*, London: Forced Marriage Unit Online. Available HTTP: <http://www.fco.gov.uk/resources/en/pdf/travel-living-abroad/when-things-go-wrong/fm-disability-guidelines> (accessed 25 February 2012).

HM Government (2011) *No Health Without Mental Health: A Cross-Government Mental Health Outcomes Strategy for People of All Ages*, London: DH. Online. Available HTTP: <http://www.dh.gov.uk/en/Publicationsandstatistics/Publications/PublicationsPolicyAndGuidance/DH_123766> (accessed 25 February 2012).

Holland, S. (2010) 'Looked after children and the ethic of care', *British Journal of Social Work*, 40: 1664–80.

Hollis, M. and Howe, D. (1987) 'Moral risks in social work', *Journal of Applied Philosophy*, 4: 123–32.

Hollis, M. and Howe, D. (1990) 'Moral risks in the social work role: a response to Macdonald', *British Journal of Social Work*, 20: 547–52.

Home Affairs Select Committee (2011) *Forced Marriage: Eighth Report of Session 2010-12*, HC 880, London: TSO. Online. Available HTTP: <http://www.publications.parliament.uk/pa/cm201012/cmselect/cmhaff/880/880.pdf> (accessed 25 February 2012).

Home Office (1990) *Crime, Justice and Protecting the Public*, Cm 965, London: HMSO.

Home Office (2010) *Child Sex Offender Disclosure Scheme Guidance Document*, London: Home Office. Online. Available HTTP: <http://www.homeoffice.gov.uk/publications/crime/disclosure-scheme-guidance/> (accessed 25 February 2012).

Home Office (2011a) *Domestic Violence Disclosure Consultation*, London: Home Office. Online. Available HTTP: <http://www.homeoffice.gov.uk/publications/about-us/consultations/domestic-violence-disclosure/> (accessed 25 February 2012).

Home Office (2011b) *Forced Marriage Consultation*, London: Home Office. Online. Available HTTP: <http://www.homeoffice.gov.uk/publications/about-us/consultations/forced-marriage/> (accessed 25 February 2012).

House of Commons Health Committee (2012) *Social Care. Fourteenth Report of Session 2010-12*, HC 1583, London: TSO. Online. Available HTTP: <http://www.parliament.uk/business/committees/committees-a-z/commons-select/health-committee/publications/> (accessed 25 February 2012).

Houston, S. (2003) 'Establishing virtue in social work: a response to McBeath and Webb', *British Journal of Social Work*, 33: 819-24.

Houston, S. (2011) 'Engaging with the crooked timber of humanity: value pluralism and social work', *British Journal of Social Work*, advance access.

Howe, D. (1992) 'Child abuse and the bureaucratisation of social work', *Sociological Review*, 40: 491-508.

HPC (Health Professions Council) (2008) *Standards of Conduct, Performance and Ethics*, London: HPC. Online. Available HTTP: <http://www.hpc-uk.org/aboutregistration/standards/standardsofconductperformanceand ethics> (accessed 25 February 2012).

Hudson, B. (2003) *Understanding Justice: An Introduction to Ideas, Perspectives and Controversies in Modern Penal Theory*, 2nd edn, Buckingham: Open University Press.

Hugman, R. (2005) *New Approaches in Ethics for the Caring Professions*, Basingstoke: Palgrave Macmillan.

Ife, J. (2008) *Human Rights and Social Work: Towards Rights-Based Practice*, revised edition, Cambridge: Cambridge University Press.

IFSW and IASSW (International Federation of Social Workers and International Association of Schools of Social Work) (2001) *International Definition of Social Work*, Berne, Switzerland: IFSW and IASSW. Online. Available HTTP: <http://www.ifsw.org/f38000032.html> (accessed 25 February 2012).

IFSW and IASSW (2004) *Ethics in Social Work: Statement of Principles*, Berne, Switzerland: IFSW and IASSW. Online. Available HTTP: <http://www.ifsw.org/f38000032.html> (accessed 25 February 2012).

Iwaniec, D., Donaldson, T. and Allweis, M. (2004) 'The plight of neglected children: social work and judicial decision-making, and management of neglect cases', *Child and Family Law Quarterly*, 16: 423-36.

JCHR (Joint Committee on Human Rights) (2008) *A Life Like Any Other: Human Rights of People with Learning Disabilities. Seventh Report of Session 2007-08*, House of Commons and House of Lords JCHR, HC 73-I, HL 40-I, London: TSO. Online. Available HTTP: <http://www.publications.parliament.uk/pa/jt200708/jtselect/jtrights/40/40i.pdf> (accessed 25 February 2012).

Johns, R. (2011) *Using the Law in Social Work*, 5th edn, Exeter: Learning Matters.

Jones, H. and Jones, K. (2010) *Hannah's Choice*, London: Harper Collins.

Judiciary for England and Wales (2008) *Public Law Outline: Guide to Case Management for Public Law Proceedings*, London: MoJ. Online. Available HTTP: <http://www.justice.gov.uk/guidance/protecting-the-vulnerable/care-proceedings-reform.htm> (accessed 25 February 2012).

Kant, I. (1785) *The Foundation of the Metaphysics of Morals*. Translated by T. K. Abbott (1934), London: Longmans Green and Co. Online. Available HTTP: <http://www.gutenberg.org/ebooks/5682> (accessed 25 February 2012).

Katz, I., Corlyon, J., La Placa, V. and Hunter, S. (2007) *The Relationship Between Parenting and Poverty*, York: Joseph Rowntree Foundation. Online. Available HTTP: <http://www.jrf.org.uk/sites/files/jrf/parenting-poverty.pdf> (accessed 25 February 2012).

Kemshall, H. and Wood, J. (2008) 'Public protection in practice: multi-agency public protection arrangements (MAPPA)', in Clark, C. and McGhee, J. (eds) *Private and Confidential: Handling Personal Information in the Social and Health Services*, Bristol: Policy Press.

Kemshall, H. and Wood, J. (2010) *Child Sex Offender Review (CSOR) Public Disclosure Pilots: A Process Evaluation*, Home Office Research Report 32, London: Home Office. Online. Available HTTP: <http://webarchive.national archives.gov.uk/20110218135832/rds.homeoffice.gov.uk/rds/pdfs10/horr32c.pdf> (accessed 25 February 2012).

King, M. and Trowell, J. (1992) *Children's Welfare and the Law: The Limits of Legal Intervention*, London: Sage.

Laird, S. (2010) *Practical Social Work Law: Analysing Court Cases and Inquiries*, Harlow: Pearson Education.

Laming, H. (2003) *The Victoria Climbié Inquiry Report*, Cm. 5370, London: TSO. Online. Available HTTP <http://www.dh.gov.uk/en/Publicationsandstatistics/Publications/PublicationsPolicyAndGuidance/DH_40086 54> (accessed 25 February 2012).

Laming, H. (2009) *The Protection of Children in England: A Progress Report*, HC 330, London: TSO. Online. Available HTTP: <https://www.education.gov.uk/publications/eOrderingDownload/HC-330.pdf> (accessed 25 February 2012).

Lavalette, M. (ed.) (2011) *Radical Social Work Today: Social Work at the Crossroads*, Bristol: Policy Press.

Law Commission (2008) *Tenth Programme of Law Reform*, Law Com 311, London: TSO. Online. Available HTTP: <http://www.justice.gov.uk/lawcommission/docs/lc311_10th_Programme.pdf> (accessed 25 February 2012).

Law Commission (2010) *Adult Social Care: A Consultation Paper*, Consultation Paper 192, London: The Law Commission. Online. Available HTTP: <http://www.justice.gov.uk/lawcommission/areas/adult-social-care.htm> (accessed 25 February 2012).

Law Commission (2011) *Adult Social Care: Final Report*, Law Com 326, London: TSO. Online. Available HTTP: <http://www.justice.gov.uk/lawcommission/areas/adult-social-care.htm> (accessed 25 February 2012).

LCD (Lord Chancellor's Department) (2002) *Scoping Study on Delay in Children Act Cases*, London: LCD.

LCD (2003) *Protocol for Judicial Case Management in Public Law Children Act Cases*, London: LCD.

Lloyd, L. (2006) 'A caring profession?' The ethics of care and social work with older people', *British Journal of Social Work*, 36(7): 1171-85.

Long, L-A., Roche J. and Stringer, D. (eds) (2010) *The Law and Social Work: Contemporary Issues for Practice*, 2nd edn, Basingstoke: Palgrave Macmillan.

Lorenz, W. (1994) *Social Work in a Changing Europe*, London: Routledge.

Lukes, S. (2005) *Power: A Radical View*, 2nd edn (first edn 1974), London: Macmillan.

Lyons, B. (2010) 'Dying to be responsible: adolescence, autonomy and responsibility', *Legal Studies*, 30(2): 257-78.

McBeath, G. and Webb, S. (2002) 'Virtue ethics and social work: being lucky, realistic and doing one's duty', *British Journal of Social Work*, 32: 1015-36

McDonald, A. (2007) 'The impact of the UK Human Rights Act 1998 on decision making in adult social care in England and Wales', *Ethics and Social Welfare*, 1(1): 76-94.

McDonald, A. (2010) 'The impact of the 2005 Mental Capacity Act on social workers' decision making and approaches to the assessment of risk', *British Journal of Social Work*, 40: 1229-46.

Macdonald, G. (1990a) 'Allocating blame in social work', *British Journal of Social Work*, 20: 525-46.

Macdonald, G. (1990b) 'Moral risks?: a reply to Hollis and Howe', *British Journal of Social Work*, 20: 553-56.

McGhee, J. and Clark, C. (2008) 'Introduction' in Clark, C. and McGhee, J. (eds) *Private and Confidential: Handling Personal Information in the Social and Health Services*, Bristol: Policy Press.

MacIntyre, A. (1985) *After Virtue: A Study in Moral Theory*, 2nd edn, London: Duckworth.

McKeigue, B. and Beckett, C. (2004) 'Care proceedings under the 1989 Children Act: rhetoric and reality', *British Journal of Social Work*, 34: 831-49

McKeigue, B. and Beckett, C. (2010) 'Squeezing the toothpaste out of the tube: will tackling court delay result in pre-court delay in its place?', *British Journal of Social Work*, 40: 154-69.

McLaren, H. (2007) 'Exploring the ethics of forewarning: social workers, confidentiality and potential child abuse disclosures', *Ethics and Social Welfare*, 1(1): 22-40.

McLaughlin, K. (2005) 'From ridicule to institutionalization: anti-oppression, the state and social work', *Critical Social Policy*, 25(3): 133-48.

McLaughlin, K. (2010) 'The social worker versus the General Social Care Council: an analysis of Care Standards Tribunal hearings and decisions', *British Journal of Social Work*, 40: 311-27.

Macpherson, W. (1999) *The Stephen Lawrence Inquiry: Report of an Inquiry by Sir William Macpherson of Cluny*, Cm. 4262-I, London: TSO. Online. Available HTTP: <http://www.archive.official-documents.co.uk/document/cm 42/4262/4262.htm> (accessed 25 February 2012).

McSherry, D. (2004) 'Which came the first, the chicken or the egg? Examining the relationship between child neglect and poverty', *British Journal of Social Work*, 43: 727-33.

McSherry, D. (2007) 'Understanding and addressing "the neglect of neglect": why are we making a mole-hill out of a mountain?', *Child Abuse and Neglect*, 31: 607-14.

Mandelstam, M. (2011) *Safeguarding Adults at Risk of Harm: A Legal Guide for Practitioners*, SCIE Report 50, London: SCIE. Online. Available HTTP: <http://www.scie.org.uk/publications/reports/report50.pdf> (accessed 25 February 2012).

Mantle, G. and Backwith, D. (2011) 'Poverty and social work', *British Journal of Social Work*, 40: 2380-97.

Marshall, T. (1999) *Restorative Justice: An Overview*, London: Home Office. Online. Available HTTP: <http://library.npia.police.uk/docs/homisc/occ-resjus.pdf> (accessed 25 February 2012).

Masson, J. (2006) 'The Climbié Inquiry: context and critique', *Journal of Law and Society*, 33(2): 221-43.

Masson, J. (2010) 'A new approach to care proceedings', *Child and Family Social Work*, 15: 369-79.

Masson, J., Pearce, J. and Bader, K., with Joyner, O., Marsden, J. and Westlake, D. (2008) *Care Profiling Study*, London: Ministry of Justice. Online. Available HTTP: <http://www.justice.gov.uk/publications/docs/care-profiling-study.pdf> (accessed 25 February 2012).

Meagher, G. and Parton, N. (2004) 'Modernising social work and the ethics of care', *Social Work and Society*, 2(1): 10-27.

Mencap (2007) *Death by Indifference*, London: Mencap. Online. Available HTTP: <http://www.mencap.org.uk/node/5863> (accessed 25 February 2012).

Mencap (2012) *Death by Indifference: 74 Deaths and Counting. A Progress Report 5 Years On*, London: Mencap. Online. Available HTTP: <http://www.mencap.org.uk/74deaths> (accessed 25 February 2012).

Michael, J. (2008) *Healthcare For All, Report of Independent Inquiry into Access to Healthcare for People with Learning Disabilities*. Online. Available HTTP: <http://www.dh.gov.uk/en/Publicationsandstatistics/Publications/PublicationsPolicyAndGuidance/DH_099255> (accessed 25 February 2012).

Miles, J. (2001) '*Z and Others v United Kingdom*; *TP and KM v United Kingdom*: human rights and child protection', *Child and Family Law Quarterly*, 431-54.

Mill, J. S. (1859) *On Liberty*. Online. Available HTTP: <http://www.utilitarianism.com> (accessed 25 February 2012).

Mill, J. S. (1861) *Utilitarianism*. Online. Available HTTP: <http://www.utilitarianism.com> (accessed 25 February 2012).

Mnookin, R. and Kornhauser, L. (1979) 'Bargaining in the shadow of the law: the case of divorce', *Yale Law Journal*, 88: 950-97.

MoJ (Ministry of Justice) (2007) *Confidence and Confidentiality: Openness in the Family Courts - A New Approach*, London: TSO. Online. Available HTTP: <http://www.justice.gov.uk/docs/consult-family-courts.pdf> (accessed 25 February 2012).

MoJ (2008a) *Deprivation of Liberty Safeguards: Code of Practice to Supplement the Main Mental Capacity Act 2005 Code of Practice*, Norwich: TSO. Online. Available HTTP: <http://www.dh.gov.uk/prod_consum_dh/groups/dh_digitalassets/@dh/@en/documents/digitalasset/dh_087309.pdf> (accessed 25 February 2012).

MoJ (2008b) *Family Justice in View*, Cm 7502, Norwich: TSO. Online. Available HTTP: <http://www.official-documents.gov.uk/document/cm75/7502/7502.pdf> (accessed 25 February 2012).

MoJ (2009a) *Rights and Responsibilities: Developing Our Constitutional Framework*, Cm. 7577, Norwich: TSO. Online. Available HTTP: <http://www.official-documents.gov.uk/document/cm75/7577/7577.pdf> (accessed 25 February 2012).

MoJ (2009b) *MAPPA Guidance 2009, Version 3.0*, London: MoJ. Online. Available HTTP: <http://www.justice.gov.uk/downloads/guidance/prison-probation-and-rehabilitation/public%20protection%20manual/10004894MAPPAGuidance_2009_Version3.pdf> (accessed 25 February 2012).

MoJ (2009c) *One Year On: The Initial Impact of the Forced Marriage (Civil Protection) Act 2007 in its First Year of Operation*, London: MoJ. Online. Available HTTP: <http://www.justice.gov.uk/publications/docs/one-year-on-forced-marriage-act.pdf> (accessed 25 February 2012).

MoJ (2010) *Breaking the Cycle: Effective Punishment, Rehabilitation and Sentencing of Offenders*, Cm 7972, Norwich: TSO. Online. Available HTTP: <http://www.justice.gov.uk/consultations/docs/breaking-the-cycle.pdf> (accessed 25 February 2012).

MoJ (2011a) *Breaking the Cycle: Government Response*, Cm 8070, Norwich: TSO Online. Available HTTP: <http://www.justice.gov.uk/downloads/consultations/breaking-the-cycle-government-response.pdf> (accessed 25 February 2012).

MoJ (2011b) *Provisional Figures Relating to Offenders Serving Indeterminate Sentence for Public Protection (IPPs)*, London: MoJ. Online. Available HTTP: <http://www.justice.gov.uk/downloads/publications/statistics-and-data/mojstats/provisional-ipp-figures.pdf> (accessed 25 February 2012).

MoJ (2011c) *Family Courts Information Pilot November 2009-December 2010*, London: MoJ. Online. Available HTTP: <http://www.justice.gov.uk/downloads/publications/policy/moj/family-courts-information-pilot.pdf> (accessed 25 February 2012).

MoJ and DfE (2012) *The Government Response to the Family Justice Review: A System With Children and Families at its Heart*, Cm 8273, London: MoJ. Online. Available HTTP: <https://www.education.gov.uk/publications/standard/publicationDetail/Page1/CM-8273> (accessed 6 February 2012).

MoJ, Crown Prosecution Service, Department for Education, Department of Health and Welsh Assembly Government (2011) *Achieving Best Evidence in Criminal Proceedings: Guidance on Interviewing Victims and Witnesses, and Guidance on Using Special Measures*, 3rd edn, London: MoJ. Online. Available HTTP: <http://www.cps.gov.uk/legal/assets/uploads/files/Achieving%20Best%20Evidence%20in%20Criminal%20Proceedings.pdf> (accessed 25 February 2012).

Morgan, C., Dazzan, P., Morgan, K., Jones, P., Harrison, G., Leff, J., Murray, R. and Fearon, P., on behalf of the AESOP Study Group (2006) 'First episode psychosis and ethnicity: initial findings from the AESOP study', *World Psychiatry*, 5(1): 40-6.

Munro, E. (2007) 'Confidentiality in a preventive child welfare system', *Ethics and Social Welfare*, 1(1): 41-55.

Munro, E. (2010) *The Munro Review of Child Protection, Part One: A Systems Analysis*, London: DfE. Online. Available HTTP: <http://www.education.gov.uk/munroreview/> (accessed 25 February 2012).

Munro, E. (2011a) *The Munro Review of Child Protection, Interim Report: The Child's Journey*, London: DfE. Online. Available HTTP: <http://www.education.gov.uk/munroreview/> (accessed 25 February 2012).

Munro, E. (2011b) *The Munro Review of Child Protection, Final Report: A Child-Centred System*, London: DfE. Online. Available HTTP: <http://www.education.gov.uk/munroreview/> (accessed 25 February 2012).

National End of Life Care Programme (2010) *Supporting People to Live and Die Well: A Framework for Social Care at the End of Life*, Leicester: National End of Life Care Programme. Online. Available HTTP: <http://www.endoflifecareforadults.nhs.uk/publications/supporting-people-to-live-and-die-well-a-framework> (accessed 25 February 2012).

National Equality Panel (2010) *An Anatomy of Economic Inequality in the UK - Summary Report of the National Equality Panel*, London: Government Equalities Unit. Online. Available HTTP: <http://webarchive.national archives.gov.uk/20110608160754/http://www.equalities.gov.uk/national_equality_panel/publications.aspx> (accessed 25 February 2012).

NIMHE (National Institute for Mental Health in England) (2003) *Inside Outside: Improving Mental Health Services for Black and Minority Ethnic Communities*, Leeds: NIMHE. Online. Available HTTP: <http://www.dh. gov.uk/prod_consum_dh/groups/dh_digitalassets/@dh/@en/documents/digitalasset/dh_4019452.pdf> (accessed 25 February 2012).

NIMHE (2008) *Mental Health Act 2007: New Roles*, Leeds: NIMHE. Online. Available HTTP: <http://www.nmhdu. org.uk/silo/files/mental-health-act-2007–new-roles.pdf> (accessed 25 February 2012).

NIMHE (2009) *The Legal Aspects of the Care and Treatment of Children and Young People with Mental Disorder: A Guide for Professionals*, Leeds: NIMHE. Online. Available HTTP: <http://www.nmhdu.org.uk/silo/files/ publication-cyp-legal-guide-jan-2009.pdf> (accessed 25 February 2012).

NMHDU (2010) *Race Equality Action Plan: a Five Year Review*, London: DH. Online. Available HTTP: <http:// www.nmhdu.org.uk/silo/files/race-equality-action-plan-a-five-year-review.pdf> (accessed 25 February 2012).

Noddings, N. (2003) *Caring: A Feminine Approach to Ethics and Moral Education*, 2nd edn, Berkeley: University of California Press (first edition 1984).

Nottingham City Safeguarding Children Board (2009) *Report Regarding Issues of Consent in Relation to Baby K*, Nottingham: Nottingham City Council. Online. Available HTTP: <http://www.mynottingham.gov.uk/index. aspx?articleid=5089> (accessed 25 February 2012).

Orwell, G. (1949) *Nineteen Eighty-Four: A Novel*, London: Secker and Warburg.

Parker, P. (2009) *Professional Boundaries in Social Work: A Qualitative Study*, Report to the General Social Care Council, London: Witness. Online. Available HTTP: <http://www.gscc.org.uk/cmsFiles/Publications/GSCC_ Professional_Boundaries_Full_Report_2009.pdf> (accessed 25 February 2012).

Parrott, L. (2006) *Values and Ethics in Social Work Practice*, Exeter: Learning Matters.

Parsons, T. (1954) 'A sociologist looks at the legal profession' in *Essays in Sociological Theory*, (revised edition), New York: Free Press.

Parton, N. (1985) *The Politics of Child Abuse*, London: Macmillan.

Parton, N. (1991) *Governing the Family: Child Care, Child Protection and the State*, London: Macmillan.

Parton, N. (1998) 'Risk, advanced liberalism and child welfare: the need to rediscover uncertainty and ambiguity', *British Journal of Social Work*, 28: 5-27.

Parton, N. (2004) 'From Maria Colwell to Victoria Climbié: reflections on public inquiries into child abuse a generation apart', *Child Abuse Review*, 13(2): 80-94.

Parton, N. (2009) 'Challenges to practice and knowledge in child welfare social work: from the "social" to the "informational"?', *Children and Youth Services Review*, 31(7): 715-21.

Payne, M. (2006) *What is Professional Social Work?*, 2nd edn, Bristol: BASW/Policy Press.

PCAW (Public Concern at Work) (2011) *Speaking Up for Vulnerable Adults: What the Whistleblowers Say*, London: PCAW. Online. Available HTTP: <http://www.pcaw.co.uk/files//news_attachments/Speaking%20up%20for %20vulnerable%20adults,%20what%20the%20whistleblowers%20say,%20PCAWApril2011.pdf> (accessed 25 February 2012).

Peck, M. (2011) *Patterns of Reconviction Among Offenders Eligible for Multi-Agency Public Protection Arrangements (MAPPA)* Ministry of Justice Research Series 6/11, London: MoJ. Online. Available HTTP: <http://www.justice.gov.uk/downloads/publications/research-and-analysis/moj-research/patterns- reconviction-mappa.pdf> (accessed 25 February 2012).

Pemberton, C. (2012a) 'Family court plans "risk miscarriages of justice"', *Community Care*, 9 February. Online. Available HTTP: <http://www.communitycare.co.uk/Articles/09/02/2012/117973/family-courts-plans-risk- miscarriages-of-justice.htm> (accessed 25 February 2012).

Pemberton, C. (2012b) 'Record child referrals push social workers to breaking point', *Community Care*, 9 February. Online. Available HTTP: <http://www.communitycare.co.uk/Articles/09/02/2012/117972/record-child-referrals-push-social-workers-to-breaking-point.htm> (accessed 25 February 2012).

Pickford, J. and Dugmore, P. (2012) *Youth Justice and Social Work*, 2nd edn, London: Sage/Learning Matters.

Preston-Shoot, M. (2010) 'On the evidence for viruses in social work systems: law, ethics and practice', *European Journal of Social Work*, 13(4): 465-82.

Preston-Shoot, M. (2011) 'On administrative evil-doing within social work policy and services: law, ethics and practice', *European Journal of Social Work*, 14(2): 177-94.

PRT (Prison Reform Trust) (2007) *Indefinitely Maybe: How the Indeterminate Sentence for Public Protection is Unjust and Unsustainable*, London: PRT. Online. Available HTTP: <http://www.prisonreformtrust.org.uk/Portals/0/Documents/Indefinitely%20Maybe%20-%20IPP%20briefing.pdf> (accessed 25 February 2012).

Rawls, J. (1999) *A Theory of Justice*, revised edition, Oxford: Oxford University Press (first edition 1971).

Razack, S. (2004) 'Imperilled Muslim women, dangerous Muslim men and civilised Europeans: legal and social responses to forced marriages', *Feminist Legal Studies*, 12(2): 129-74.

RCVP (Riots, Communities and Victims Panel) (2011) *5 Days in August: An Interim Report on the 2011 English Riots*, London: RCVP. Online. Available HTTP: <http://riotspanel.independent.gov.uk/> (accessed 25 February 2012).

Read, J. and Clements, L. (2004) 'Demonstrably awful: the right to life and the selective non-treatment of disabled babies and young children', *Journal of Law and Society*, 31(4): 482-509.

Reder, P. and Duncan, S. (2003) 'Understanding communication in child protection networks', *Child Abuse Review*, 12: 82-100.

Reith, M. and Payne, M. (2009) *Social Work in End-of-Life and Palliative Care*, Bristol: Policy Press.

Rhodes, M. (1986) *Ethical Dilemmas in Social Work Practice*, Milwaukee, Wis.: Family Service America (originally published Boston, MA: Routledge and Kegan Paul).

Richardson, G. (2004) 'Impact studies in the United Kingdom' in Hertogh, M. and Halliday, S. *Judicial Review and Bureaucratic Impact: International and Interdisciplinary Perspectives*, Cambridge: CUP.

Richardson, S. and Asthana, S. (2006) 'Inter-agency information sharing in health and social care services: the role of professional culture', *British Journal of Social Work*, 36: 657-69.

Sandel, M. (2009) *Justice: What's the Right Thing to Do?* London: Penguin.

SAP (Sentencing Advisory Panel) (2008) *Consultation Paper on Principles of Sentencing for Youths*, London: SAP. Online. Available HTTP: <http://www.banksr.co.uk/images/Guidelines/Advisory%20Panel%20Consultation%20Papers/The_principles_of_sentencing_for_youths.pdf> (accessed 25 February 2012).

SCIE (Social Care Institute for Excellence) (2011) *Deprivation of Liberty Safeguards: At a Glance Guide 43*, London: SCIE. Online. Available HTTP: <http://www.scie.org.uk/publications/ataglance/ataglance43.asp> (accessed 25 February 2012).

SCMH (Sainsbury Centre for Mental Health) (2002) *Breaking the Circles of Fear: A Review of the Relationship Between Mental Health Services and African and Caribbean Communities*, London: SCMH. Online. Available HTTP: <http://www.centreformentalhealth.org.uk/pdfs/Breaking_the_Circles_of_Fear.pdf> (accessed 25 February 2012).

Scourfield, P. (2007) 'Social care and the modern citizen: client, consumer, service user, manager and entrepreneur', *British Journal of Social Work*, 37: 107-22.

Sen, A. (2009) *The Idea of Justice*, Cambridge, Mass.: Harvard University Press.

Sevenhuijsen, S. (2000) 'Caring in the third way: the relation between obligation, responsibility and care in *Third Way* discourse', *Critical Social Policy*, 20: 5-37.

Sewell, H. (2009) *Working with Ethnicity, Race and Culture in Mental Health: A Handbook for Practitioners*, London: Jessica Kingsley

Seymour, R. and Seymour, C. (2011) *Courtroom and Report Writing Skills for Social Workers*, 2nd edn, Exeter: Learning Matters.

SGC (Sentencing Guidelines Council) (2008) *Overarching Principles: Assaults on Children and Cruelty to a Child, Definitive Guideline*, London: Sentencing Guidelines Secretariat. Online. Available HTTP: <http://sentencing council.judiciary.gov.uk/docs/web_Overarching_principles_assaults_on_children_and_cruelty_to_a_child.pdf> (accessed 25 February 2012).

Sherman, L. and Strang, H. (2007) *Restorative Justice: The Evidence*, London: The Smith Institute. Online. Available HTTP: <http://www.restorativejustice.org.uk/resource/restorative_justice_the_evidence__professor_lawrence_ sherman_and_dr_heather_strang/> (accessed 25 February 2012).

Sinclair, I. and Corden, J. (2005) *A Management Solution to Keeping Children Safe: Can Agencies On Their Own Achieve What Lord Laming Wants?* York: Joseph Rowntree Foundation. Online. Available HTTP: <http://www.jrf.org.uk/sites/files/jrf/1859353940.pdf> (accessed 25 February 2012).

Squires, P. (2006) 'New Labour and the politics of antisocial behaviour', *Critical Social Policy*, 26: 144-68.

Squires, P. (ed) (2008) *ASBO Nation: The Criminalisation of Nuisance*, Bristol: Policy Press.

Steel, N., Blakeborough, L. and Nicholas, S. (2011) *Supporting High-Risk Victims of Domestic Violence: A Review of Multi-Agency Risk Assessment Conferences (MARACs)*, Home Office Research Report 55, London: Home Office. Online. Available HTTP: <http://www.homeoffice.gov.uk/publications/science-research-statistics/research-statistics/crime-research/horr55/> (accessed 25 February 2012).

Stevenson, O. (1988) 'Law and social work education: a commentary on the "Law Report"', *Issues in Social Work Education*, 8(1): 37-45.

Stevenson O. (2007) *Neglected Children and their Families*, 2nd edn, Oxford: Blackwell.

Sunkin, M., Calvo, K. and Platt, L. (2008) *Does Judicial Review Influence the Quality of Local Authority Services?* ESRC Public Services Programme Discussion Paper 0801. Online. Available HTTP: <http://www.public services.ac.uk/wp-content/uploads/dp0801_final.pdf> (accessed 25 February 2012).

Swain, P. (1989) 'From Carney to Cleveland ... to Chinkapook and Cottles Bridge or lawyer and social worker ... Can the marriage work?', *Journal of Social Welfare and Family Law*, 11: 229-34.

Swain, P. (2006) 'A camel's nose under the tent? Some Australian perspectives on confidentiality and social work practice', *British Journal of Social Work*, 36: 91-107.

SWRB (Social Work Reform Board) (2010) *Building a Safe and Confident Future: One Year On - Progress Report from the Social Work Reform Board*, London: SWRB. Online. Available HTTP <https://www.education.gov.uk/publications/standard/publicationdetail/page1/dfe-00601-2010> (accessed 25 February 2012).

SWTF (Social Work Task Force) (2009a) *First Report of the Social Work Task Force*, May 2009, London: SWTF. Online. Available HTTP <http://dera.ioe.ac.uk/1911/1/FirstReport.pdf> (accessed 25 February 2012).

SWTF (2009b) *Facing Up to the Task: The Interim Report of the Social Work Task Force*, July 2009, London: SWTF. Online. Available HTTP <http://webarchive.nationalarchives.gov.uk/+/www.dh.gov.uk/en/SocialCare/DH_098 322> (accessed 25 February 2012).

SWTF (2009c) *Building a Safe, Confident Future: The Final Report of the Social Work Task Force*, December 2009, London: SWTF. Online. Available HTTP <http://webarchive.nationalarchives.gov.uk/+/www.dh.gov.uk/en/SocialCare/DH_098322> (accessed 25 February 2012).

Taylor, R. (2007) 'Reversing the retreat from Gillick? R (Axon) v Secretary of State for Health', *Child and Family Law Quarterly*, 19(1): 81

This is Nottingham (2009) 'Mother threw baby at social worker', 14 February. Online. Available HTTP: <http://www.thisisnottingham.co.uk/Mother-threw-baby-social-worker/story-12260551-detail/story.html> (accessed 25 February 2012).

Thompson, N. (1992) *Existentialism and Social Work*, Aldershot: Avebury.

Thompson, N. (2000) 'Existentialist practice' in Stepney, P. and Ford, D. (eds) *Social Work Theory and Method*, Lyme Regis: Russell House.

Thompson, N. (2008) 'Existentialist ethics: from Nietzche to Sartre and beyond', *Ethics and Social Welfare*, 2(1): 10-23.

Thompson, N. (2011) *Promoting Equality: Working with Diversity and Difference*, 3rd edn, Basingstoke: Palgrave Macmillan.

Tonry, M. (ed) (2011) *Why Punish? How Much? A Reader on Punishment*, Oxford: Oxford University Press.

Travers, M. (2010) *Understanding Law and Society*, Abingdon: Routledge.

Travis, A. (2011) 'Kenneth Clarke down, prison population up', *The Guardian*, 21 June. Online. Available HTTP: <http://www.guardian.co.uk/commentisfree/2011/jun/21/kenneth-clarke-sentencing-reforms> (accessed 25 February 2012).

Tronto, J. (1993) *Moral Boundaries: A Political Argument for an Ethic of Care*, London: Routledge.

UN (United Nations) (2004) *The Rule of Law and Transitional Justice in Conflict and Post-Conflict Societies*, S/2004/616, New York: UN Security Council. Online. Available HTTP: <http://www.un.org/en/ruleoflaw/index.shtml> (accessed 25 February 2012).

Unison (2011) *Duty of Care Handbook*, London: Unison. Online. Available HTTP: <http://www.unison.org.uk/healthcare/dutyofcare/index.asp> (accessed 25 February 2012).

Wacks, R. (2009) *Understanding Jurisprudence: An Introduction to Legal Theory*, 2nd edn, Oxford: Oxford University Press.

WAG (Welsh Assembly Government) (2008) *Mental Health Act 1983 Code of Practice for Wales*, Cardiff: WAG. Online. Available HTTP: <http://www.wales.nhs.uk/sites3/Documents/816/Mental%20Health%20Act%201983%20Code%20of%20Practice%20for%20Wales.pdf> (accessed 25 February 2012).

Ward, H., Brown, R., Westlake, D. and Munro, E. (2010) *Infants Suffering, or Likely to Suffer, Significant Harm: A Prospective Longitudinal Study*, DfE Research Brief RB053, London: DfE. Online. Available HTTP: <https://www.education.gov.uk/publications/RSG/AllPublications/Page1/DFE-RB053> (accessed 25 February 2012).

Ward, L. (2008) 'Reflections on the ethics of participation in secret filming', *Ethics and Social Welfare*, 2(1): 100-3.

Watt, N. (2011) '124 Sure Start centres have closed since coalition took power', *Guardian Society*, 14 November. Online. Available HTTP: <http://www.guardian.co.uk/society/2011/nov/14/sure-start-centre-closures-coalition> (accessed 25 February 2012).

Weinberg, M. (2010) 'The social construction of social work ethics: politicizing and broadening the lens', *Journal of Progressive Human Services*, 21: 32-44.

White, R., Broadbent, G. and Brown, K. (2009) *Law and the Social Work Practitioner*, 2nd edn, Exeter: Learning Matters

Williams, F. (2001) 'In and beyond New Labour: towards a new political ethics of care', *Critical Social Policy*, 21: 467-93.

Williams, J. (2008) *Child Law for Social Work*, London: Sage.

Williams, J. (2010) 'Remedies' in Long, L-A., Roche J. and Stringer, D. (eds) *The Law and Social Work: Contemporary Issues for Practice*, 2nd edn, Basingstoke: Palgrave Macmillan.

Wood, J. and Kemshall, H., with Maguire, M., Hudson, K., and McKenzie, J. (2007) *The Operation and Experience of Multi-Agency Public Protection Arrangements*, London: Home Office. Online. Available HTTP: <http://www.caerdydd.ac.uk/socsi/resources/MAPPA1207.pdf> (accessed 25 February 2012).

Index